Longman Housecraft Series

Food and Nutrition

Longman Housecraft Series

This series brings to the study of Home Economics
an approach which is both practical and humane.
Teachers and pupils will find that the material for study
is related to our lives today in a meaningful way without
neglecting the historical world-wide context. They will also
find that these books give the study its true
significance in human affairs, the series as a whole
being designed to implement the more liberal thinking
in Home Economics associated with the Certificate of
Secondary Education.

Phyllis Davidson	THE FAMILY IN THE COMMUNITY
Joan Dixon	HOUSES AND HOUSING
Brenda Piper	FIBRES AND FABRICS
Rena Cloke	DESIGN

Food and Nutrition

Barbara Hammond

TEACHER'S DIPLOMA OF BATTERSEA POLYTECHNIC TRAINING
COLLEGE OF DOMESTIC SCIENCE
FORMERLY DEPUTY PRINCIPAL AND PRINCIPAL LECTURER IN
COOKERY AT BATTERSEA TRAINING COLLEGE OF
DOMESTIC SCIENCE

Illustrated by Rowan Barnes-Murphy

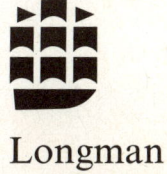

Longman

LONGMAN GROUP LIMITED
London
*Associated companies, branches and representatives
throughout the world*

© Longman Group Limited 1975

First published 1975

ISBN 0 582 22157 9

Filmset by Photoprint Plates Limited, Rayleigh, Essex
Printed in Great Britain by
Lowe & Brydone (Printers) Ltd, Thetford, Norfolk

Foreword

Home Economics with a wide concept of family life has now, for most of us, replaced Domestic Science with its sub-divisions into Cookery. Housewifery and Laundrywork. In this wider treatment the subjects rightly merge into one another and all are fitted into the pattern of living in families and in society. Food, however, is so important to the life of every individual from infancy to old age that it deserves special attention from the points of view of nutrition, and consequently health, and of a family's economic and social life.

In this book it is hoped to relate the study of food to the way we live and also to open the doors of Home Economics even wider so that it may take a look at food in the world outside the home. In touching on how and where some foods are produced and processed the book aims at showing the link between other school subjects and the study of food.

The horizon is widened still further to include a glimpse of pressing world food problems today.

Above all it is intended to encourage further reading and further investigation into some of the many aspects of a study of food. It is a starter—not the whole meal!

Acknowledgements

Photographs are reproduced by permission of the following:

Barnaby's Picture Library, p. 23 bottom (photo Pierre Berger), p. 101 top left. Batchelor's Foods Ltd, p. 53 bottom. Birds Eye Foods Ltd, p. 54 British Egg Information Service, pp. 78 top and bottom, 79 top and bottom. Campbell Soups Ltd, p. 53 top. Daily Mirror—Slimming and Nutrition Magazine, pp. 33 top, right and centre. FAO, pp. 104, 108 (photo P. Pittet), 110 (photo G. Bavagnoli), 111 top and bottom (photos by courtesy of the Public Health Department of Iran), 113 (photo G. Bavagnoli), 114 (photo G. Tortoli), 115 (photo D. Mason), 117 (photo Y Nagata) 119 top, 119 bottom, 120 top (photo G. Tortoli), 121 (photo G. Mason). Eastern Electricity, pp. 57 bottom left and right, 58 bottom right. Findus Ltd, p. 92 centre. Milk Marketing Board, pp. 67 bottom, 83, 86 top. Poultry World, pp. 75 top and bottom. Spectrum Colour Library, pp. 23 centre (photo Tony Boxall FRPS), 90 bottom. Homer Sykes, pp. 11, 21, 23 centre right, 27 centre left, 27 bottom left, 28 top left, top right, centre left, centre right, bottom left, bottom right, 32 top left, centre left, bottom left, 39, 40, 41 bottom left, bottom right, 43 top left, 46, 47, 48, 49, 61 left, 62 top left and right. Photographic Library, Tate and Lyle Refineries Ltd, p. 101 bottom left. John Topham Ltd, pp. 14, 67 top right, bottom right, 69, 70 bottom left and right, 71 bottom right, 74 bottom, 77 bottom right, 81, 82, 85 bottom left and right, 86 bottom left and right, 90 top, 91 bottom left and right, 92 bottom right, 102. Thomas A. Wilkie, FRPS, AIBP, p. 67 top left.

Contents

Acknowledgements

The author gratefully acknowledges the encouragement and advice of Miss B. W. Merson, Principal Lecturer in Food and Nutrition and of Mrs A. Lerwill, Librarian, both of Battersea College of Education.

1st Course   Fish Remove.

Transparancy Soup.

Pigeon. Compot.   Frica'd. Chickens.

Flamis.

Lamb Ears Forc'd.   Codicums like little Turkeys.

French Pye   Pork Griskins.   Fricand Veal.

Kidney Beans.   Brocoli &c.

Boil'd Turkey.   Bottl'd. Peas.   Mod Turtle.   Sallad.   Small Ham.

Green Peas & Kidneys in Rice   Larded Oysters   House Lamb.   Ox Pallets   Sweet Breads Ala Royal.

Hornade of Rabbits   Beef Olives.   Duck Alonade.

Hare Soup.

Part of an 18th century
Gourmet's dinner menu.

1 The Food We All Need

CHOOSING

How important is food? We know that we must eat to live but there are several other answers to the question. Some people, *gourmets,* are fond of food for its own sake and rank its importance very high while others are far more occupied with other interests and activities so that, to them, food is little more than a tiresome interruption in the day's work. Between these two extremes most of us enjoy our food and find meals pleasant occasions at which we can meet and talk to our family or our friends while we eat food that we like. Few of us eat only to live.

Think of a dinner that you really enjoy eating and write the menu down. Write down several if you like.

Now think carefully what led you to choose as you did. Did you choose dishes you know well because you often have them at home; did you choose foods that are popular or fashionable with your group of friends or were you really thoughtful and practical so that you considered what food you could afford and could buy in your local shops at the present time? In other words were you guided by traditions of your family and the part of the country in which you live or by fashion or by practical considerations of economy and the availability of foods?

THE RIGHT DIET

All three are quite usual ways of choosing foods to make up a meal or the day's meals, that is the *diet.* When we go shopping and look at the vast array of foodstuffs on display in a supermarket or even in the little shops round the corner the choice is truly bewildering. Some guideline is therefore needed to lead us to a sensible choice of diet and the safest guideline is a knowledge of the foods which our bodies need and the particular work each kind of food can carry out in keeping us healthy.

Presumably we all want to feel lively and well and to look our best and, although even a perfect diet cannot endow us with fabulous beauty, a good diet can go a long way towards giving us clear, healthy skin, glossy hair, strong teeth and well-proportioned bodies. The right diet

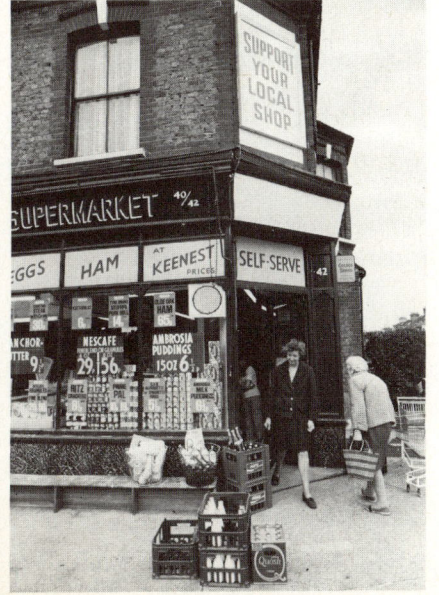

11

can, furthermore, help us to enjoy just being alive and give us energy to enjoy all our activities of work and play.

The foods that we need in our diet to give us this alive look and this feeling of enjoyment of living can be divided into groups according to the particular part they play in keeping us healthy. We should eat something from each group (with one group excepted) at every meal if possible and certainly every day.

FIVE GROUPS OF FOODS

Group I. For growth and repair

Milk — At least one pint a day until you are over eighteen.

Cheese, Eggs, Meat, including ham and bacon, Fish — An average helping from each of two or three of these items every day.

If you are a vegetarian, nuts, pulses (that is peas, beans and lentils), and cereals (such as wheat, oats, barley or rye) will replace meat and fish and perhaps the whole group if you are a strict vegetarian *(a vegan)*.

Group II. For general health and liveliness

Oranges, lemon juice, grapefruit (fresh, not bottled 'squash')
Green vegetables, green salads
Purple, red or orange coloured vegetables and fruit
Any other vegetables or fruit — An average helping from each of two, or better three, items every day, if possible using all lines and using the items raw if they are edible raw.

Group III. For concentrated energy and warmth

Margarine, butter and other fats and oils — Spread on bread or used in cooking

Group IV. For energy and warmth and to satisfy hunger

Bread
Potatoes
Cereals
Chocolate
Honey and jam
Pastry
Sugar, biscuits and cakes — Most meals should include one or two of these—they are important in the diet but not every one of them is needed every day. It is important to be sparing with the items in the last four lines.

Group V. For health and growth

Herrings, fresh or canned
Mackerel and sprats
Sardines
Salmon, fresh, frozen or canned
Liver

A helping once a week of any one of them will be enough, but if you like them of course have them more often.

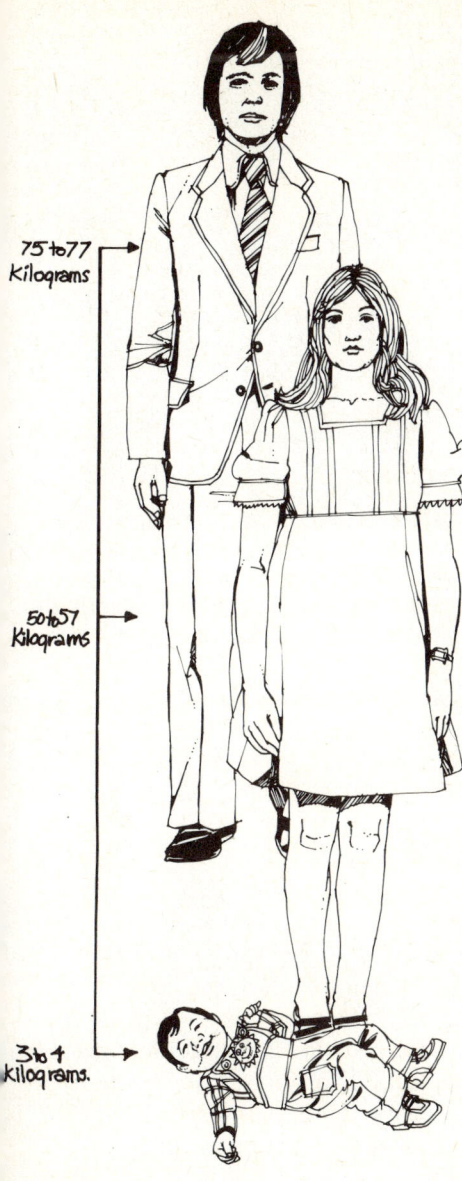

75 to 77
kilograms

50 to 57
kilograms

3 to 4
kilograms.

Each group contains certain foods which have an important part to play in the work of keeping us in full health. We shall find that some groups overlap with others. This, you will readily see, makes planning a diet easier.

Group I includes the foods which mainly provide material for growth and for keeping the whole body in a good state of repair. Food for growth is obviously particularly necessary for children. Just think what a lot of growing a person has to do in the first sixteen to twenty years of his or her life. A baby has to develop from a small, soft, helpless individual, weighing only 3 to 4 kilograms, to a tall, strong man weighing 75 to 77 kilograms or to a fully developed woman weighing 50 to 57 kilograms and able to have babies herself. Only the right amount of building food (see group I) during babyhood and childhood can ensure that the baby grows as strong and healthy as its inheritance allows. In chapter 2 the special needs of babies and children will be considered.

Even when the human body is fully grown and fully developed the building foods are still needed because the millions of minute cells, which make up the highly complicated whole structure and which carry out the many different processes which keep it alive and active, are all the time wearing themselves away and needing to be replaced.

Now list the processes which you know that your body has to carry out during the twenty-four hours of the day.

PROTEIN

The only foods which can build the body structure and repair it as it wears away with use are those which contain *protein* which is the name given to the most important *nutrient* in our diet. All living things contain protein otherwise they could not grow, but in some, such as green leafy plants, the amount is so small that an enormous amount would have to be eaten to provide enough material

13

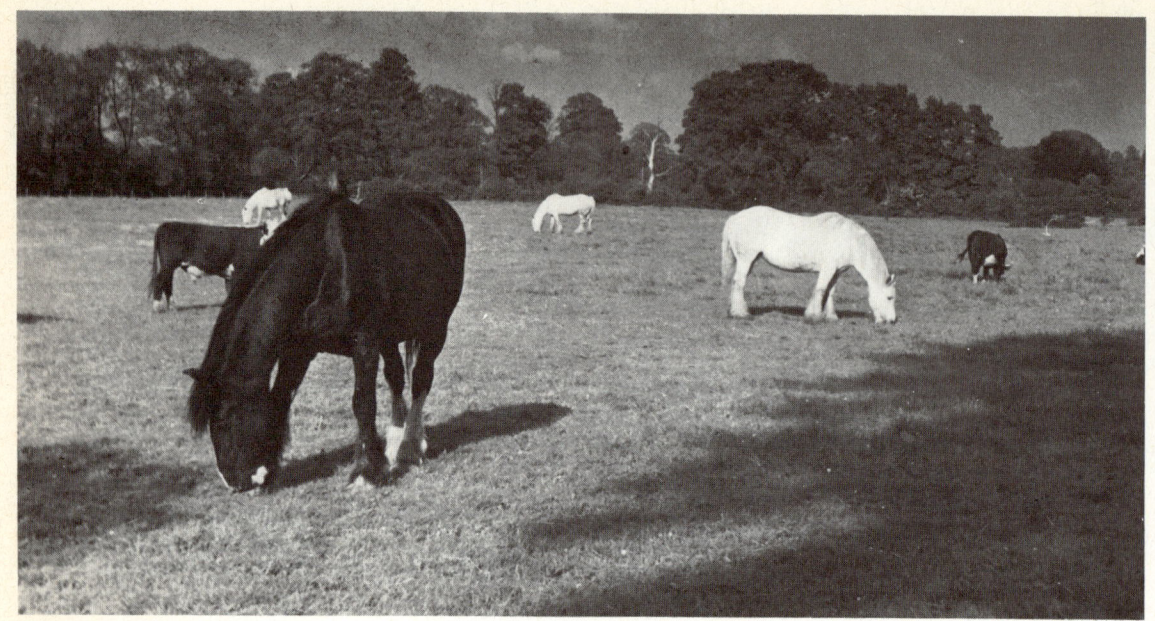

for growth. If you consider the animals that live mainly on green, leafy foods aren't they rather different in shape from us? Can you think why?

For us human beings the protein foods which are converted most easily to the protein of our own bodies are those from animal sources although the parts of plants designed especially for growth, that is their seeds, are also useful. Proteins are all built up of groups of units called *amino acids*, of which there are some twenty-three in different proteins. Eight of these amino acids are esential to the growth and repair of all human bodies, with another two which children need. Most animal proteins contain all these essential amino acids in more or less the right proportions for human needs whereas vegetable proteins all lack one or more of them. The proteins which contain all the essential amino acids in suitable proportions are said to be of *high biological value* and those that have few are of *low biological value*. In human diet a mixture of animal and vegetable proteins provides the best and most convenient supply of growth material though it is possible to live perfectly well on a mixture of vegetable proteins as vegetarians do.

Groups II, III and V contain foods which are vitally important for keeping our bodies in full health. The nutrients for which they are valuable are *minerals* and *vitamins*.

Minerals

Minerals are amply provided in a reasonably mixed diet. They are needed by the body for four main purposes:
to help in the formation and maintenance of bones and teeth;
to keep the blood and other body fluids in the right condition to carry food around the body;
to help in the repair of cells, in this they supplement proteins; and to help generally in the absorption and use of other foods.

Nineteen different minerals are needed by our bodies—too many to list here and in fact many of them are needed in very small amounts—in fact only traces of some are needed. The three important ones that we must make sure we include in our diet are calcium, phosphorus and iron.
Calcium is needed for bones, teeth and also hair and nails to be strong and healthy. The best sources are:

Milk and cheese	
Canned fish if the bones are eaten	groups I and V
Herring	
White bread	group IV
Wholemeal bread	
Egg	group I
Cabbage, turnip and lettuce	group II

Phosphorus works with calcium for bone and teeth formation, helps in the use of food for energy and keeps body fluids in the right condition. The best sources are:

Cheese	group I
Oatmeal	group IV
Liver and kidney	
Egg	groups I and IV
Milk	
White bread	group IV
Cabbage and potato	groups II and IV

Calcium and phosphorus can only work with each other and vitamin D (see later) helps them in their work.
Iron gives blood its red colour and is necessary for carrying

oxygen from the lungs to all parts of the body. The best sources are:

Liver	group V
Chocolate and cocoa ⎫	group IV
Wholemeal bread ⎭	
Egg ⎫	group I
Meat, especially corned beef ⎭	
Green peas	group II
White bread ⎫	group IV
Raisins ⎭	
Green vegetables	group II
Potato	group IV

From the above lists you can see that if food is chosen from all the groups there should be enough of these three minerals in the diet.

Vitamins

Vitamins, like minerals, are numerous, they are found in minute amounts in foods but nevertheless they are of very great importance to the healthy working of every part of our bodies. They can be divided into two main groups: *fat soluble* and *water soluble* and they are given letters to identify them as well as rather complicated names. The letters are easier to remember.

The fat soluble vitamins are A and D, the important pair, with E and K only needed in the very tiny amounts found in milk, wheat and in some green vegetables.

Vitamin A is needed for the growth of children; for controlling the way eyes see light and for keeping the moist surfaces of eyes, nose, throat and other moist areas such as bronchial tubes healthy. If we do not have enough vitamin A we are more than normally likely to catch colds; if we eat plenty in the autumn any extra can be stored in the liver for use during the winter months.

The best sources of this vitamin are animal foods, fats and fat fish, with supplementary sources in dark green, orange and red fruit and vegetables.

Animal sources of vitamin A

Halibut and cod liver oil ⎫	
Ox liver ⎭	group V
Butter ⎫	group III
Margarine ⎭	

Herring, sardines, salmon   group V

Eggs
                         } group I
Milk

Vegetable sources of Vitamin A (carotene)

Carrot
Spinach
Watercress
Tomato   } group II
Cabbage
Green peas
Dried apricots and prunes

The vitamin A in vegetables is in a different form from that in animal foods, we need twice as much of it and it has to be converted to the animal form by our digestive processes: this conversion is most complete if the vegetable is eaten with some fat or oil. The vegetable form is called carotene, can you see why?

Vitamin D is needed to form strong bones and teeth and to do this it must combine with the right amount of calcium and phosphorus. It is especially important to babies, small children and expectant mothers. Babies who do not have enough vitamin D usually have rickets. Our skin can manufacture vitamin D if it is exposed to sunlight—so children who get plenty of sunlight on their bodies can do with less vitamin D in their food. British babies and children need vitamin D for a large part of the year and the most usual form in which it is given is as halibut or cod liver oil, but only in medically prescribed doses.

The best sources of vitamin D

Halibut and cod liver oil	
Herring and canned salmon	group V
Margarine	group III
Eggs	group I
Liver	group V
Butter from summer milk	group III
Cheese from summer milk	} group I
Milk in the summer	

Vitamins A and D are added to margarine in larger proportions than are usually found in butter. There is little vitamin D in milk and therefore in butter and cheese unless cows have grazed in sunny weather.

The water soluble vitamins are B and C. B is really a large

17

group of similar vitamins often found in the same foods. There are some thirteen of them which are given B numbers and scientific names. The three vitamins of this *B complex* which are most commonly named are:

B1 or thiamine;

B2 or riboflavin;

B3 or niacin.

In general the B complex helps the growth of children, keeps skin healthy, it releases the energy from the foods we eat from group IV and in general it helps us to keep calm and good tempered. One vitamin of this complex, B12 helps to prevent some kinds of anaemia.

The best sources of vitamin B

Dried brewer's yeast	B1, B2, B3	
Pork	B1, B3	group I
Wholemeal bread	B1, B3	
White bread	B1, B3	group IV
Oatmeal	B1	
Potato	B1, B3	group IV
Milk	B1, B2 (only a little), B12	
Liver	B2, B3, B12	
Eggs	B2, B12	group I
Fish	B3, B12	
Beef	B2, B3, B12	

From this list you can see that with a good mixed diet it is easy to make sure of a supply of B complex, there is a little of B1 and B3 in most vegetables especially green peas and if you are in doubt about the supply, dried yeast will certainly provide plenty.

Vitamin C (also called ascorbic acid) is found only in fruit and vegetables, and in liver and kidney which contain a little. Unfortunately some of the best sources are usually expensive and, equally unfortunately, as it cannot be stored by the body, some source of it must be eaten every day. It is also easily lost during the cooking of fruit and green vegetables.

Vitamin C is lost from green vegetables:

by oxidation if they are stale, crushed or bruised;

by dissolving into water if they are soaked, or cooked in too much water;

completely destroyed if they are overcooked or kept hot for more than a few minutes.

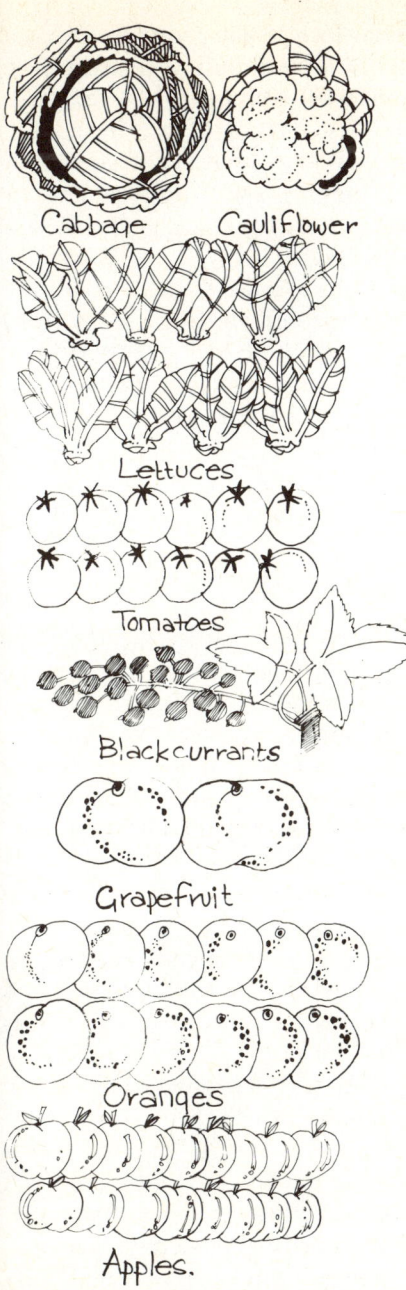

Cabbage   Cauliflower

Lettuces

Tomatoes

Blackcurrants

Grapefruit

Oranges

Apples.

There is roughly the same amount of vitamin C in each of these groups.

Overcooked green vegetables not only lose all vitamin C they also taste and look horrible.

To make sure that vitamin C is not lost

Use all vegetables while they are fresh and crisp;
use vegetables raw in salad when possible;
cook them for as short a time and in as little water as possible;
use the cooking-water in gravy or soup the same day;
NEVER keep green vegetables hot.

Vitamin C is another vitamin that aids growth in children; it enables the body to absorb iron from food; it can aid the healing of wounds and fractures and it helps to keep the gums healthy. Without enough vitamin C people can get an unpleasant disease called scurvy. Sailors suffered from this in the days of sailing ships, which were often at sea for several months without fresh fruit and vegetables. Long ago some sea captain found that limes (fruit like a small lemon) could cure his men, and limes were often part of the sailors' diet thereafter.

The best sources of vitamin C (all from group II)

FRUITS	Blackcurrants
	Other summer soft fruits
	Oranges and lemons
	Grapefruit
VEGETABLES	Brussels sprouts and cabbage
	Cauliflower
	Watercress
	Spinach
	Potatoes, but only when they are new
	Lettuces, a little.

Of popular fruits apples have very little (their best use is for cleaning teeth at the end of a meal). The popular salad of lettuce and tomato does not yield very much vitamin C. You need to eat four times as much lettuce and three times as much tomato by weight to get the same amount of vitamin C as you would from an average helping of raw or properly cooked (i.e., not overcooked) sprouts, cauliflower or cabbage.

Potatoes when they are first dug as new potatoes are a good source of vitamin C but with storage the vitamin slowly diminishes so that by March they yield hardly any.

Fresh fruit and vegetables lose all their vitamin C when dried in the hot air or sun, but retain all of it when deep frozen, AFD and vacuum dried (see pp. 53, 54 for these methods). Canned fruit has less vitamin C than fresh fruit. Canned fruit has more vitamin C than fruit stewed at home because, during the canning, the fruit is cooked 'or processed' in the can after it has been sealed. Oxidation cannot take place inside the sealed can.

Canned vegetables have less vitamin C than fresh ones because vegetables (except tomatoes which are really fruit) do not contain much acid, which acts as a preservative. During canning they must be heated to a higher temperature for a longer time than fruit, and the higher temperature destroys some of the vitamin C.

FOODS FOR FUEL

Groups III and IV

In these two groups the foods are used by the body for energy. Apart from giving energy, as we have found, some of them also contain minerals and vitamins and some in group IV have useful amounts of vegetable protein. On the whole though they are the foods chiefly used by the body as fuel. As we move about, even gently, in the every-day activities of getting dressed, walking about the house, eating or just sitting we are using energy. Still more if we rush upstairs, run, play ball games, join in P.E. or do muscular work we use a great deal of energy. Even when we lie quite still, asleep, we still use energy to keep breath-ing, to keep our hearts beating, our blood circulating and our temperature at the right level. This use of energy is known as *basal metabolism*.

As we digest fuel foods they release energy, which as you probably know always produces heat so the fuel foods also keep us warm.

The two groups of fuel foods are fats and oils in group III and *carbohydrates* in group IV, that is *starch and sugar*. Starch is the fuel food in cereals and some vegetables, notably potatoes; sugar is in all foods that are naturally sweet. Both kinds of fuel food are needed in our diet.

Fats and oils are concentrated fuel foods so that quite a small amount of them can produce a lot of energy. Unless some of our energy is obtained from fat we should need to eat a rather bulky diet. Some of the fat we eat is used to form a layer of fat just under the skin which acts like a blanket to keep us warm and some is used as protective packing round important organs such as the kidneys.

Starch in food we convert to sugar as we digest it and as sugar it is carried round the body in the bloodstream to supply energy where it is needed. If we eat more starch and sugar than we can use up as energy the sugar is still further changed into fat which is stored all over the body, usually to our inconvenience.

In butter and margarine as we have noted there are important vitamins—A and D. In the starchy group, bread and potatoes contain minerals, protein and some of the B vitamins so it is important that these foods are used as part of our fuel ration. Sugar and pure starch such as corn-flour and custard powder are only fuels and the least important in the group; they are called 'empty calories' (see chapter 2).

The two groups III and IV are usually well represented in our diet and we have to remember that they are not all builders and none of them contain all the minerals and vitamins we need. On the other hand the building foods in group I, if we eat more of them than we need, can be used as fuel. This is very extravagant as they are all more expensive than those in group IV. If we eat more building food than we need and also more fuel food the digestive system can convert the protein into fat and can make us still fatter. Some fuel food should be eaten at every meal that includes protein foods so that the expensive growth and building material is not wasted.

ROUGHAGE

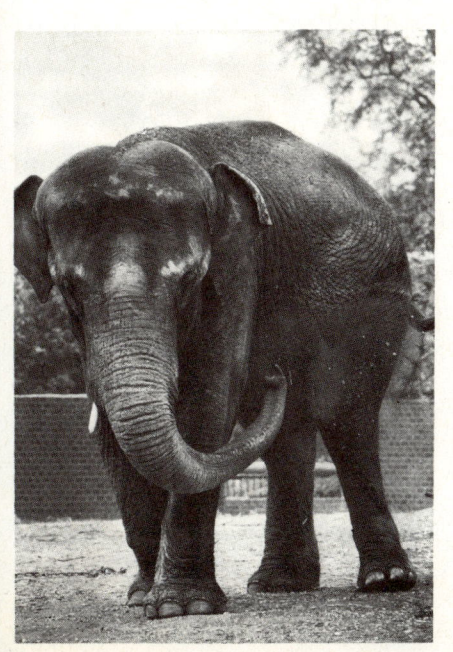

In groups II and IV, that is in most vegetable foods, the fibrous part is another kind of carbohydrate called *cellulose* which is not much use as a nutrient in our food because our digestive system cannot absorb it. It is, however, useful as 'roughage' to help us to get rid of the waste matter from food through the bowel. Herbivorous animals can munch and enjoy such cellulose foods as hay and even straw because, unlike humans, their digestive organs are designed to deal with such food.

21

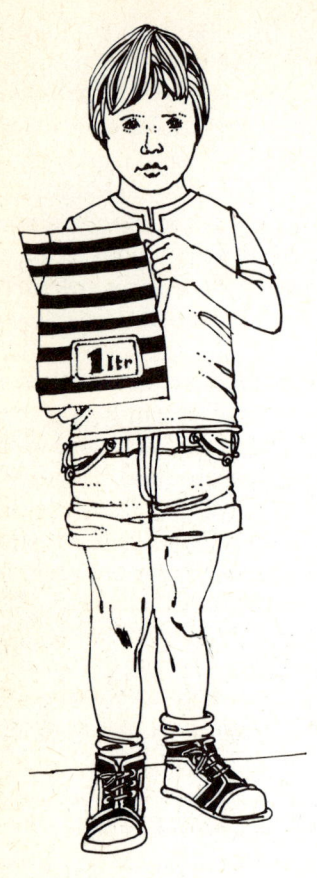

WATER

Water is another item of diet that is not a nutrient although hard water may contain useful minerals in very small amounts. We ourselves are made up of at least 60 per cent water and most of our food contains as much or more. We need water to carry digested food round the body; to keep our cooling system working by means of perspiration and to wash away in urine much soluble waste matter. We need to drink at least 1 litre (1½ to 1¾ pints) of liquid every day, in addition to the water contained in our food.

Things to do

1. Look back to the meal you thought of and check with the five food groups to see if your meal includes something from each.
2. If one group has been omitted how can you include in your meal the missing item?
3. Using the groups as guide, plan some other good meals and a whole day's meals for yourself.
4. If you have a chance cook at least one of the meals you planned and eat it with your family or friends. Listen to their criticism.
5. Make sure that you really understand any new words you have found in this chapter.

Further reading

HMSO. *Manual of Nutrition* (latest edition), Part 1, 1970.

MINISTRY OF HEALTH (Central Office of Information), Pamphlets.

MATTHEWS, W, and WELLS, D. *The Second Book of Nutrition,* Home Economics and Domestic Science Review & Flour Advisory Bureau, 1968.

WATERS, D. *Learning about Food,* Teachers' Handbook National Dairy Council, 1972.

HUTCHINS, K. C. *Food and Your Body,* National Dairy Council.

BOOTHMAN, D. B. et al. Topical Workbooks No. 5, *Food to Eat,* Longman, 1968.

EDEN VALE PAMPHLET. 'Beauty', Express Dairies Ltd.

NATIONAL DAIRY COUNCIL PAMPHLET. 'Looking Ahead', 1969.

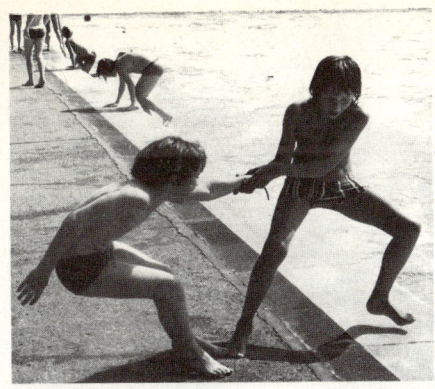

2 Food for All the Family

THE RIGHT AMOUNT

In chapter 1 we studied the groups of food from which we must choose our meals every day and the nutrients that they contain and, rather generally, why we need these nutrients. But does everyone need the same amount and the same proportions of different foods? You can probably think of differences in the appetites of different members of your own

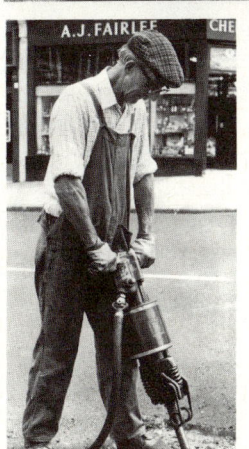
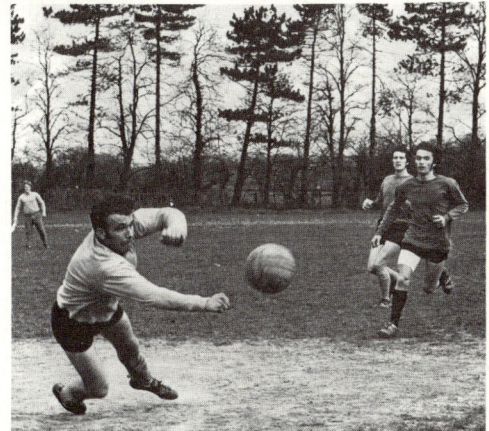
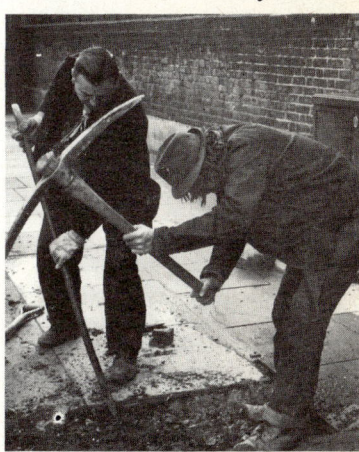

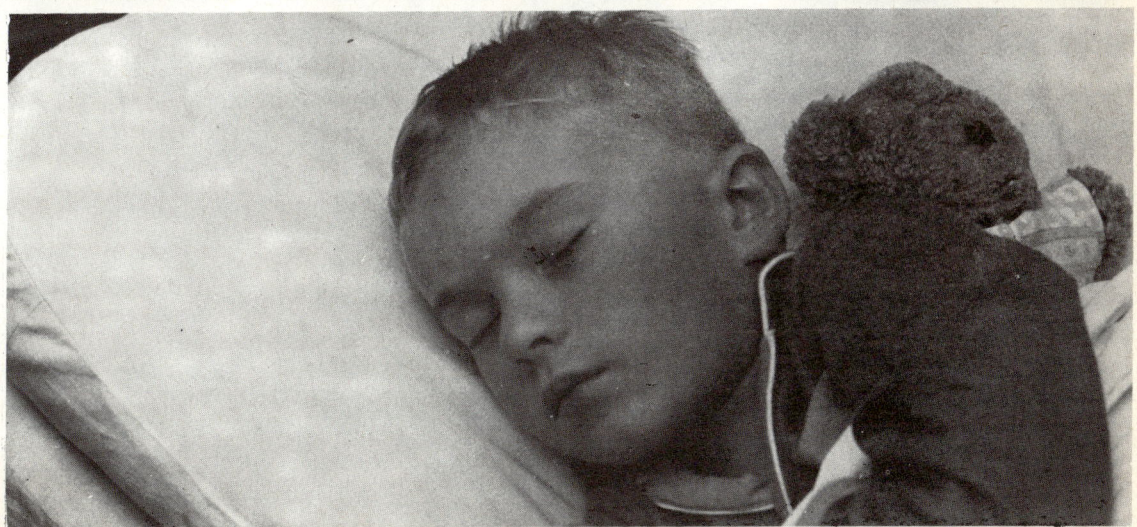

family especially if the family includes a grandparent and a young baby. It is quite right that there should be such differences because the amount and sometimes the kinds of food that people need vary with their age, the kind of work or play that they engage in and according to whether they are male or female. The size and weight of a grown up will also affect the amount of food he or she needs but not as much as will age and activity.

Approximately the right amount of food for people of different ages and occupations has been worked out by food scientists with most complicated arithmetic. They calculate the energy value of each food by measuring the heat it gives off when burnt. The amount of energy used by people of different weights carrying out various activities has also been estimated, the amount is related to the total surface area of the body. Though children are smaller than adults and therefore use less energy, their surface area in proportion to their weight is greater and therefore the amount of food they need is also proportionately greater.

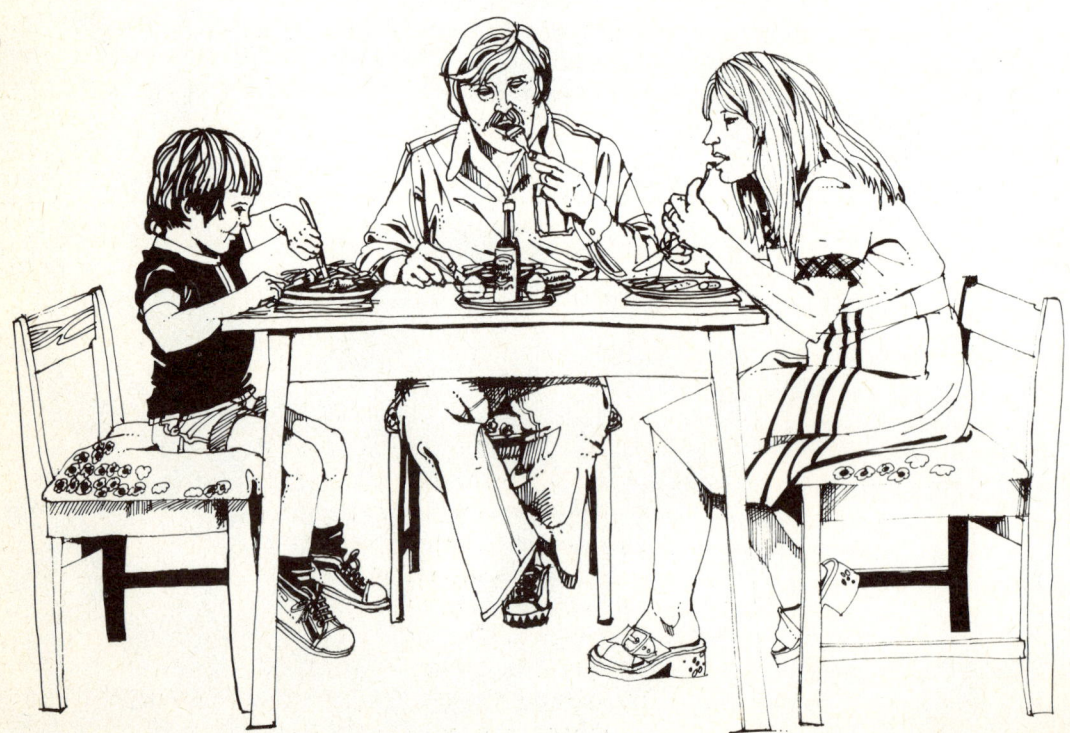

CALORIES

The energy value of food is measured in units of heat called *kilo calories* (= 1000 calories) and written *kcal*. In 1970 a new term called *Joule* for measuring units of heat was introduced, and this term will eventually replace *kcal*. 1 kcal is equal to 4·184 *kilojoules* (4·184 kJ). See Manual of Nutrition 1970 pp. 75–90. A kcal is the amount of heat needed to raise the temperature of 1 kilogram of water through one degree centigrade. If this sounds complicated just think of it simply as a unit of the fuel needed by the body.

Kcal produced by the main nutrients

1 gram fat produces about 9 kcal
   (37·6 kJ)
1 gram sugar produces about 3·75 kcal
   (15·7 kJ)
1 gram protein produces about 4 kcal
   (8·18 kJ)

fat, sugar and protein here mean *nutrients* NOT *foods*

Examples of approximate kcal value of average helpings of everyday foods.

From group I	Approx kcal	Approx kJ
Milk, ½ pt (280 ml)	200	837
Yoghurt, 5 oz (142 ml)	80	335
Cheese (Cheddar), 2 oz (57 g)	230	962
Egg, 1 standard	80–90	335–376
Meat (lean beef), raw, 4 oz (113 g)	240	1004
Bacon, 2 rashers	270	1130
Bacon (1 rasher) and 1 egg	200–15	837–899
Sausages, 2	370	1548
Cooked ham etc, 2 oz (57 g)	240	1004
Fish, 4 oz (113 g), after cooking	150	628
Fish: herrings (cooked), sardines, canned salmon, 4 oz (113 g)	250	1046
Fish fingers, 2 oz (57 g)	208	870
Fried fish, 4 oz (113 g)	225	941
Baked beans, 4 oz (113 g)	100	418
From group II		
Apple, 1	40	167
Banana, 1	35–40	146–167
Cabbage, cooked, 4 oz (113 g)	8	33

Lettuce, 2 oz (57 g)	5–6	21–25
Carrots, 4 oz (113 g)	28	117
Peas (fresh or frozen, cooked) 4 oz		
(112 g)	50	209
Canned fruits, 4 oz (113 g)	80–100	335–418
Rhubarb with sugar, 4 oz (113 g)	100–20	418–502
Orange, 1	35–40	146–167
From group III		
Margarine or butter, $\frac{1}{2}$ oz (14 g)	110	460
From group IV		
Bread large, thick slice 2 oz (57 g)	120–40	502–586
Potatoes, boiled, 4 oz (113 g)	88	368
Potatoes, fried chips, 4 oz (113 g)	260	109
	(frying adds at least 100 kcal)	
Breakfast cereal (unsweetened),		
$\frac{3}{4}$ oz (22 g)	90	376
Cake (fairly rich), 2 oz (57 g)	140	586
Chocolate, 2 oz bar (57 g)	290	1213
Sweet biscuits, 2	125	523
Sugar, 1 teaspoonful	20	84
Jam, 1 teaspoonful	15	63
Fruit pie, 4 oz (113 g), fruit 1 oz		
(28 g) pastry	250–300	1046–1255
Milk pudding, $\frac{1}{4}$ pt (140 ml) milk,		
$\frac{1}{2}$ oz (14 g) cereal	150	628
Custard, thick sauce or gravy,		
2 tbsp.	100	418
Ice cream, 5 oz (142 ml)	150	628
Coca cola, 1 can or bottle	100	418

These kcal values of foods are only important as a rough check on the total amount of food anyone eats in a day and this total will of course be made up of a mixture of foods from all the groups, in other words, from a good mixed diet. Kcal alone are not a guide to a good diet.

Next we need to know how many kcal any person needs in a day and how the amount varies for different ages and occupations.

For comparison, the daily needs of different people for kcal are roughly as follows:

		kcal	kJ
A *baby*, 1 year	about	1000–1200	4184–5021
A *small child*, 3 to 5 years	,,	1600	6694
A *child*, 12 years	,,	2300	9623
A *boy*, 15 years, normally active	,,	2800	11715
A *girl*, 15 years, normally active	,,	2300	9623
A *woman*, weighing about 8½ to 9 stone (55 kg) doing sedentary work	,,	2100	8786
doing very active work	,,	2500	10460
A *man*, weighing 10 stone (65 kg) doing sedentary work	,,	2500	10460
doing very active work	,,	3500	14644

Take a careful look at these figures and notice all the variations.

Note: For more detailed study of the daily food needs of different groups of people read *Manual of Nutrition* pp. 40–44.

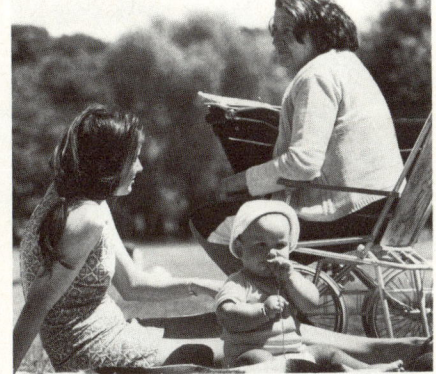

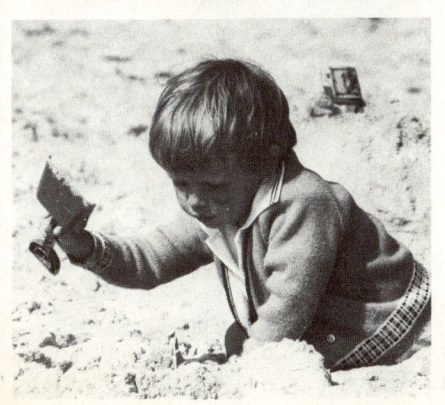

BABIES

To begin at the beginning, with a young baby it is easy to understand why he only needs a small amount of food. He is not only small but also he hasn't the strength to be very active, much as he may wriggle and kick and wave his arms. But, in fact he needs about twice as much food per kg of his weight as does a grown man. He has no teeth at first so he cannot eat solid food but he has a lot of growing to do so his food must contain plenty of food from group I (protein food). As you know, for the first few months of life the baby lives almost entirely on milk—no chewing is needed and almost all the nutrients he needs are there in the right proportions, that is in his mother's milk or in specially prepared baby food or modified cow's milk.

Almost but not quite all the nutrients are there. There will be enough building material for his rapid growth, enough fat and sugar to give him energy and to keep him warm and

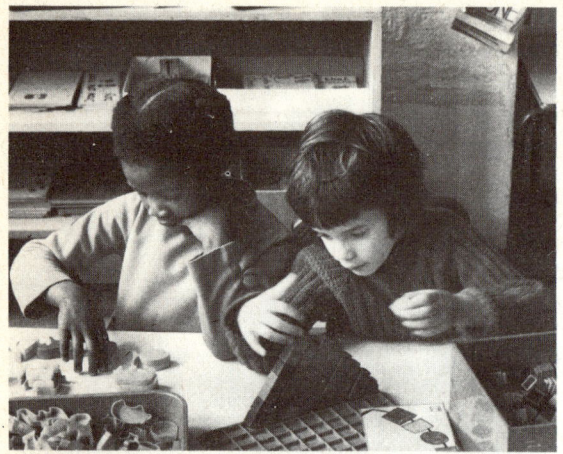
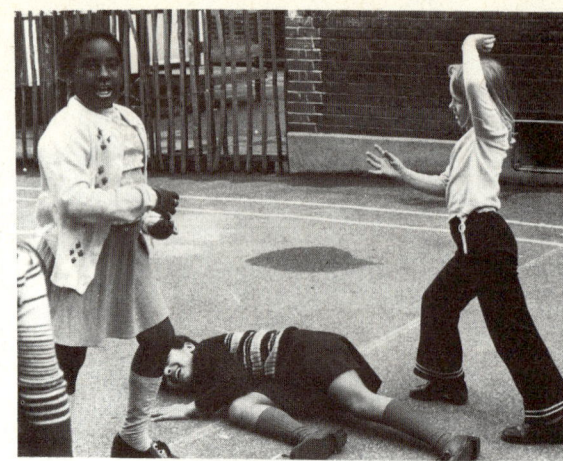
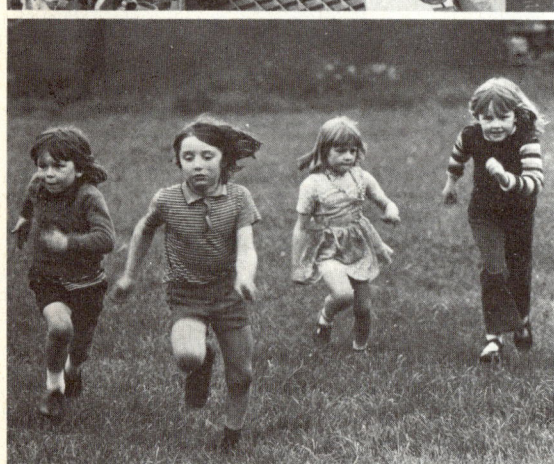
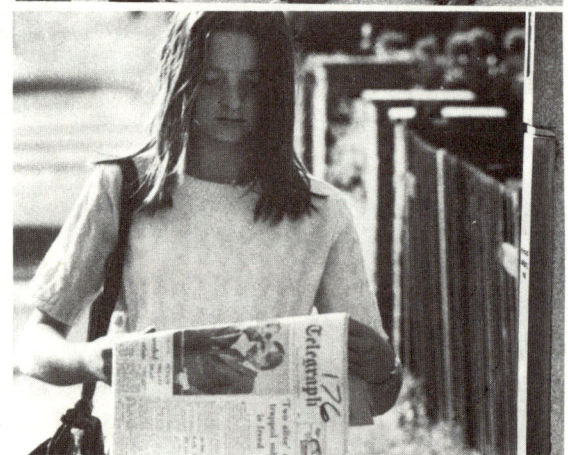
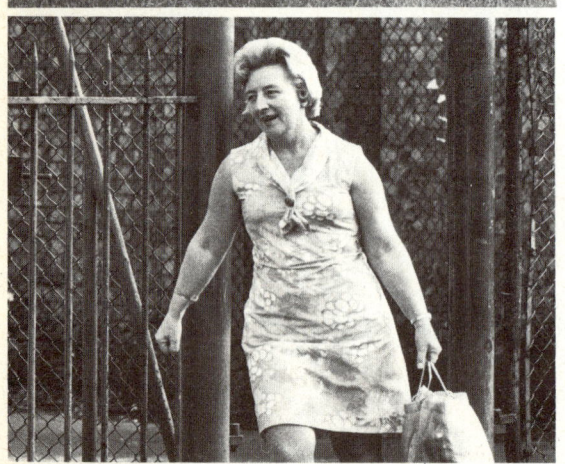
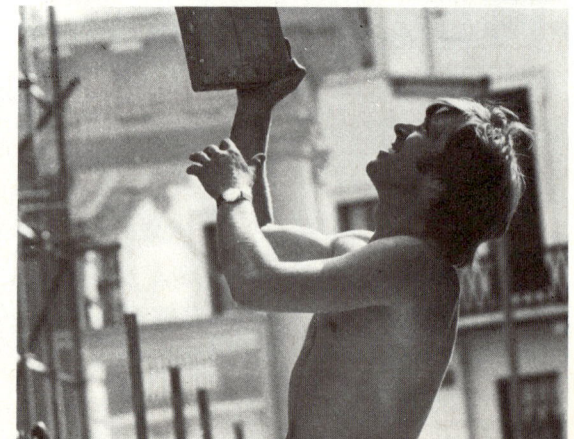

enough calcium and vitamin B to aid his growth. But there may not be enough vitamin C, and in cold, sunless weather there may not be enough vitamin D. Babies are therefore given a little orange juice and sometimes, in winter, a little cod or halibut liver oil.

Another lack as the baby gets older is iron; he is born with enough iron in his body to last him for the first few months but at about three months old he will need a little egg yolk to give him not only iron but also extra calcium and vitamins A and D and building material. It is not a good idea to give a baby extra starchy gruel until the Welfare experts or the doctor recommend it: it will only make the baby too fat and fat babies are not usually the healthiest.

As the baby grows he gets more energetic and his teeth begin to come through so he needs some solid food to bite on—still plenty of milk but he now progresses from sieved vegetables and fruit, minced meat and semi-liquid cereal mixtures to small portions of hard foods like rusks, crisp apple and solid pieces of meat or fish until, by the time he is one year old, he can eat a mixed diet almost like the rest of the family but in small helpings and still with plenty of milk. Because the baby is still small and cannot therefore eat very much at a meal it is important that the building foods (group I) and the foods containing vitamins and minerals (group II) and foods from the first three lines of group IV with the occasional helping from group V are eaten first and that sweet puddings or cakes are left till last so that he will only eat them if he is really hungry.

There are one or two important rules to follow in choosing a good diet for a baby or toddler. First, food should not be too highly flavoured or seasoned as a small child really enjoys the natural taste of foods and second, and even more important, it is mistaken kindness to give a baby very sweet foods or many sweets. Sugar and sweet, starchy foods are the greatest enemies of our teeth and, as too many of us know, decaying teeth can be painful. Although the baby's first teeth will fall out when he is six or seven the second set are already growing in the gums and if the first ones decay it is most likely that the second teeth will be of poor quality. No one really wants false teeth! Sweet and starchy foods are also the greatest contributors to over fatness; an overfat baby will probably grow into an overfat schoolchild who would probably much rather be slim and spry. Later, of

29

course, the fat child may become a fat adult and there are many disadvantages to that.

VERY YOUNG CHILDREN

As children grow older the same pattern of foods is right but of course the helpings are larger and food need not be minced or sieved. It is still important that, in any meal, the building foods and those that contain vitamins and minerals are really eaten and that the fuel-only foods are used as fillers in case the child is still hungry at the end of the main part of the meal. The building foods must still include milk—at least one pint a day. Every meal should include some hard food to give the teeth some exercise and it is an easy way of cleaning teeth at the end of a meal to eat a piece of apple or celery.

SCHOOL CHILDREN

School children are still growing fast and are using up much more energy than they did when they were smaller at home but they are still not very big and cannot eat a large amount at one meal so it is very important that their meals are not filled out too much with soft drinks or inessential foods such as packet soups and jellies. The group I and groups II, III and V foods provide the growth material that they need, always remembering that milk is still about the best growth food. Foods in group IV need more careful choice; bread, biscuits, cake, wheaten breakfast cereal and puddings made from wheat flour provide quite a useful amount of calcium, iron and vitamin B and also a little building material in addition to their value as fuel: oatmeal is rather like wheat in many ways but custard powder, pudding powders, instant whips, cornflakes (made from maize or rice) and cornflour are really only fuels and their chief use is to make milk more attractive.

If we consider the popular extras such as sweets and ice cream, one of them—chocolate, especially if it has nuts, raisins and milk in it, is a good food with plenty of iron and calcium; boiled sweets and toffees are only fun and are bad for the teeth. Ice cream also, if it is made with milk or cream (and it must be labelled as such) is quite a good food but iced lollies are only synthetic flavourings, sugar and water, they may be fun but they are not food.

TEENAGERS

As you probably noticed in the table for the 9- to 18-year-olds the total fuel need of teenage boys is greater than that of girls. This is because boys as a rule use up more energy than girls do, and also because girls usually finish growing sooner than boys. Another point you probably noticed is that boys and girls in their teens need as much food or even more food as their fathers and mothers respectively. To account for this we must realise that teenagers are still growing more or less rapidly and are also maturing into men and women.

Teenage boys and young men should rightfully have large appetites, and they usually have. When they demand or gladly accept larger helpings of building foods such as meat, bacon and eggs or cheese than any one else in the family they are not just being greedy, they really need this extra building food to complete their full growth. Only if father is doing very heavy work does he need more.

Big appetites cannot be satisfied with building foods alone. In any case these are mostly too expensive, so the fuel foods are also important; but, as for all other ages, the fuel foods should also be good sources of minerals and vitamins and should contribute some growth material. The foods in groups II and III you will remember, are extremely important for healthy growth and for keeping skin clear and eyes bright.

To help prevent the spots that worry many teenagers it is a good idea to cut down rich pastries and fried foods; to eat fruit or even raw carrot instead of sweets and to drink milk rather than 'Coke'.

Teenage girls

Girls in their teens need the same sort of diet as their brothers but in smaller amounts. As, in spite of getting hungry, they may want to keep trim figures, once they have included the necessary building foods they may satisfy hunger with more vegetables, salads or fruit, with less of the starchy foods. A special need of girls in their teens and for women up to middle age is for iron to replace the iron lost in the monthly period. Quite a good ration of iron is provided by bread, eggs, meat (especially corned beef) and chocolate and raisins are both useful extras.

ADULTS

Until old age the main variations in the food needs of adults

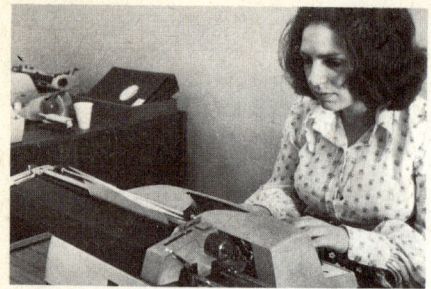

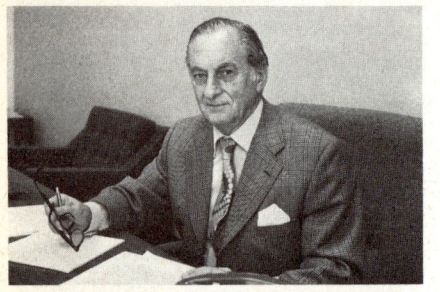

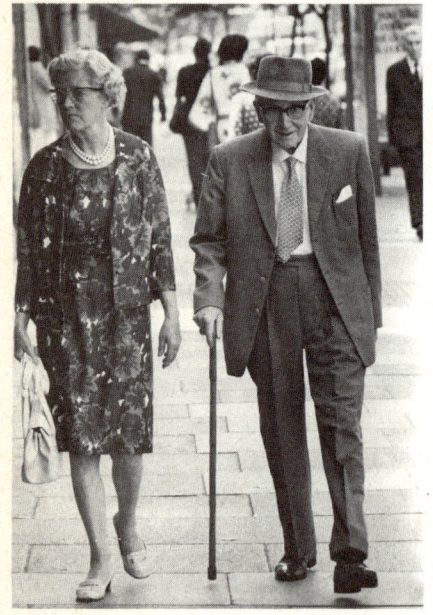

depend on the kind of work they do. Women generally need less food than men for the same kind of work. Workers in offices do not use a great deal of energy whether they are copy-typists or managing directors. They therefore need less food with a smaller proportion of fuel foods than active workers. For such *sedentary workers* vegetables, salads and fruit may replace some of the fuel foods, especially those with a high proportion of sugar. They need a helping of protein food (group I) at least twice a day with little to eat between meals—just the usual cups of tea or coffee. For sedentary workers it is most important to remember that if more kcal are supplied in food than are used up as energy for work the extra fuel is stored by the body in the form of fat and that obesity has many disadvantages and can cause various disorders in middle age. Sedentary workers fortunately are often active in their spare time.

OLD PEOPLE

The requirements of old age have not been determined but as people grow old they usually become less active and in extreme old age their weight often decreases. They probably eat less than younger adults but it is important that they should have a good supply of building foods, iron to prevent anaemia, calcium to maintain their bone structure and all vitamins. All these requirements must be met by food that they can digest. Old people sometimes find shopping and cooking difficult and tend to eat the food they find easiest to prepare such as bread and butter. Bread in itself is quite a good food but it needs additions of milk, egg, cheese and some meat and fish (canned or fresh) and these are all reasonably easy to buy and prepare. They also need foods from group II and from these an easy way to get enough vitamin C is to eat an orange a day.

SLIMMING

Having mentioned some of the disadvantages of being overweight, now let us consider how not to get too fat and how to get slim again if we do. There are many commercial products advertised nowadays that claim to have miraculous slimming powers, they are often either pills to make you lose appetite or food substitutes that make you feel as

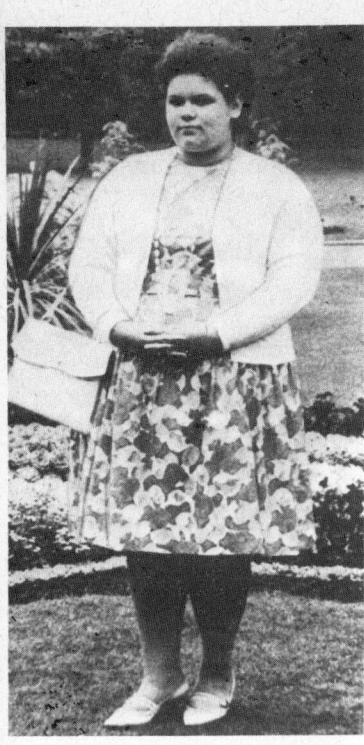
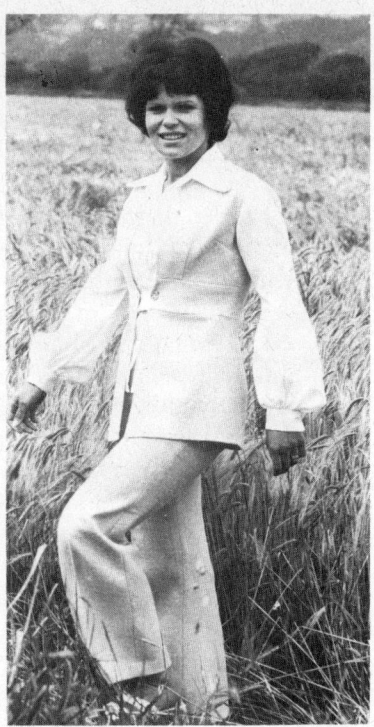

if you have had a meal when actually you have not; they certainly relieve you of some of your money but not necessarily of your excess weight. The only magic power that can help you to slim is the willpower to eat a little less, and particularly less of the tempting 'extras' such as sweets and cakes.

As well as slimming pills and biscuits a great many slimming diets are published and some of these are good, but they rather tend to advocate eating a high proportion of expensive protein foods. You can perfectly well work out your own slimming diet. To make a start decide to eat a little less altogether and then reduce the proportion of fuel foods, always remembering that you need some fuel otherwise you waste some of the building food. Among fuel foods the first to cut down is sugar and the next pure starch. The most useful way to begin slimming is to give up sweets and between-meal snacks of cake or biscuits.

Some 'crash' diets are downright dangerous when you are still growing, or at any rate young and active, because most of them leave out some essential nutrients and, though it is possible to live for a short time on one's reserves of body fat, it is immediately harmful to leave out minerals and vitamins. Only by eating a normally mixed diet is it possible to include all the essential nutrients. Crash diets are only temporary measures as a rule because it is not possible to keep to them for long. The really lasting slimming diet is one you can follow for always and that includes something from each food group.

A sensible slimming diet includes normal sized helpings of building foods, choosing lean meat and bacon, skimmed milk, cheese, including the fat fish and liver now and then and white fish. The helpings of fuel foods should be smaller than normal, choosing bread, wheat, or oatmeal products rather than cornflakes, custard powder or rice, trying to accept foods without much sugar but including a little margarine as a source of vitamin D or butter as a concentrated fuel. For the sweet course of a meal fruit is the best choice, either raw or cooked, and jelly does not add much fuel. In any slimming diet, of course, vegetables and salads are essential.

If you feel a longing for a 'little something' between meals, a very small piece of chocolate or some fruit (usually cheaper than sweets) will not add too many K calories.

Even when slimming it is not sensible to go without breakfast because during the night your body quietly uses up the food supply you gave it the day before and to start the day in a state of starvation means that you are not at your best, because your blood sugar is too low. In other words the blood has too small a source of energy to carry to any part of your body that needs it.

FAMILY MEALS

All these suggested variations of diet usually have to be provided for in meals for the whole family and tact may be needed if no member is to feel underprivileged. Generally the differences can be adjusted by varying the size of helpings; sometimes small children prefer an alternative to some unpopular food, for example raw shredded carrot or cabbage are often liked better than the cooked variety. If adults have a great liking for food quite unsuitable for young children perhaps it is kinder if they eat it after the children are in bed.

Keeping a meal hot for members of the family who come home late for the main meal is often difficult if the food is not to be spoilt. Sometimes it is possible, by taking a little more trouble, to avoid keeping it hot. It is not too difficult to cook something quickly, fresh for the latecomer; above all green vegetables are very quickly cooked and if kept hot are not only nasty but have lost all vitamin value.

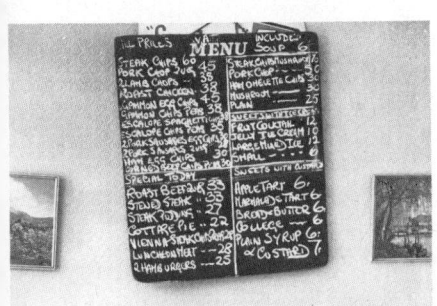

MEALS AT WORK AND AT SCHOOL

A great many people do not eat all their meals at home. Schoolchildren can have a school dinner which will be an adequate main meal; it is required to supply some of all the nutrients and about one third of the kcal needed by a teenager each day. Of course the size of helpings can be varied to suit different ages. The price of school meals is fixed by the cost of food over a wide average of prices and it has sometimes been found to be less than that of the packed meals that some children take to school. It is certainly less than the snacks they could buy outside, provided these were of equal nutritive value.

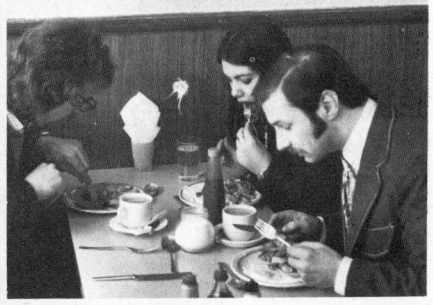

At work there are several alternatives for people who cannot be at home for one or more of their day's meals. There may be a canteen which can provide a choice of cooked meals or of snacks or the workers may buy their meals in coffee bars or restaurants outside. Workers who

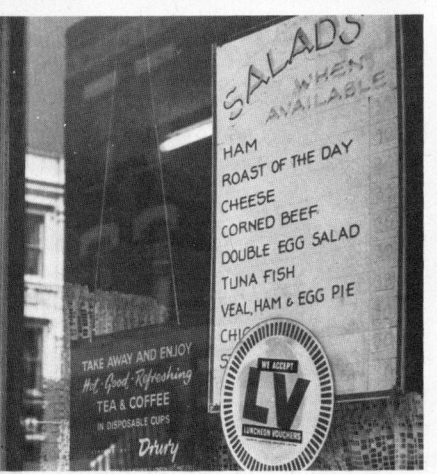

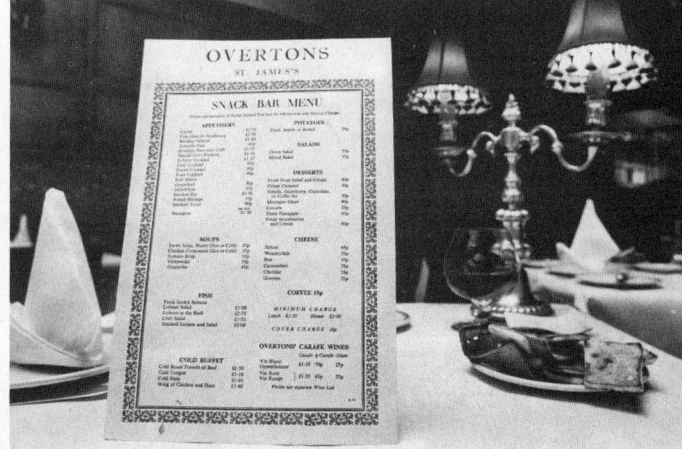

are on the move or working out of doors often must rely on a packed meal, and in some offices there is an arrangement for the staff to make a hot drink to have with their sandwiches. Now, packed lunches are traditionally made up chiefly of sandwiches but they do not have to be too much bread with a smear of fish paste or meat paste: they should make up a meal with all the food groups represented. As for the hot drinks they do not add many nutrients to the meal—a little milk in tea or coffee and in packet soups a little dried vegetable, some starch and flavouring and precious little, if any, building food.

Some firms give their employees luncheon vouchers.

Things to do

Your own diet

1. Write down accurately everything you have eaten and drunk during one day; then using the table of approximate kcal values make a rough check of your total kcal intake. Does your day's diet include the suggested helpings of all the groups in chapter 1?

2. Make up a day's menu to include all the essential nutrients that a very old couple of pensioners could afford and enjoy. Work out the cost.

3. Plan a slimming diet for someone of your own age.

4. Plan two or three packed meals that contain foods from all the first four food groups.

5. How much is a luncheon voucher worth? How can you best spend it?

6. Criticise the following snacks:

    (a) Bowl of packet soup   (b) Tomato and cheese roll
        Roll   Glass of milk
        Cream horn   Apple

    (c) Egg on chips   (d) Baked beans on toast
        cup of tea   fruit pie

    (e) Corned beef sandwich
        chocolate biscuit
        cup of coffee

    In each case is the snack a good one for a young worker in an office?
    or for a young worker doing active work?
    Note good points, bad points in each and find out the cost as far as you can.

Further reading

YUDKIN, J. *This Slimming Business,* Penguin, 1970.

EDEN VALE PAMPHLETS. 'Slimmers' Book', Express Dairies Ltd, not dated.

'Slimming Guide', *Which?*, 1972

NATIONAL DAIRY COUNCIL, *Science in Everyday Life*, (Food Experiments), 1972.

MABY, RICHARD. *Food*, Penguin Education, Connexions, 1972.

NATIONAL DAIRY COUNCIL, Set of pamphlets: 'Feeding the Under-fives'; 'Feeding the Younger Schoolchild'; 'Feeding the Older Schoolchild'.

NATIONAL DAIRY COUNCIL, *Keeping fit in retirement.*

H.M.S.O. *Recommended Intakes of Nutrients for the United Kingdom* (R.P.M.H.M.S. No. 120).

3 The Keen Shopper

BUDGETING

If you shop for food what problems do you have? Think hard for a while and imagine yourself responsible for buying all the food for a week for some particular household. You are probably at work for all or part of a five-day week so that time for shopping is limited and you also have a limited amount of money to spend.

The greatest problem is that of making the money go round. Food, although it is one of the most important items of household spending, is by no means the only thing to be paid for regularly. Rent or mortgage repayments and rates are needed for the place in which you live; this place, be it house, flat or room needs warming, lighting, cleaning and keeping in repair: you yourself and the rest of the household may have to pay fares to get to work or to school and you probably make some regular payments at work to clubs or other funds and of course you pay National Health insurance. Your personal spending on such things as clothing, shoes, toiletries, hairdressing, entertainment and holidays has to be allowed for and last, but by no means least, some money must be set aside for savings.

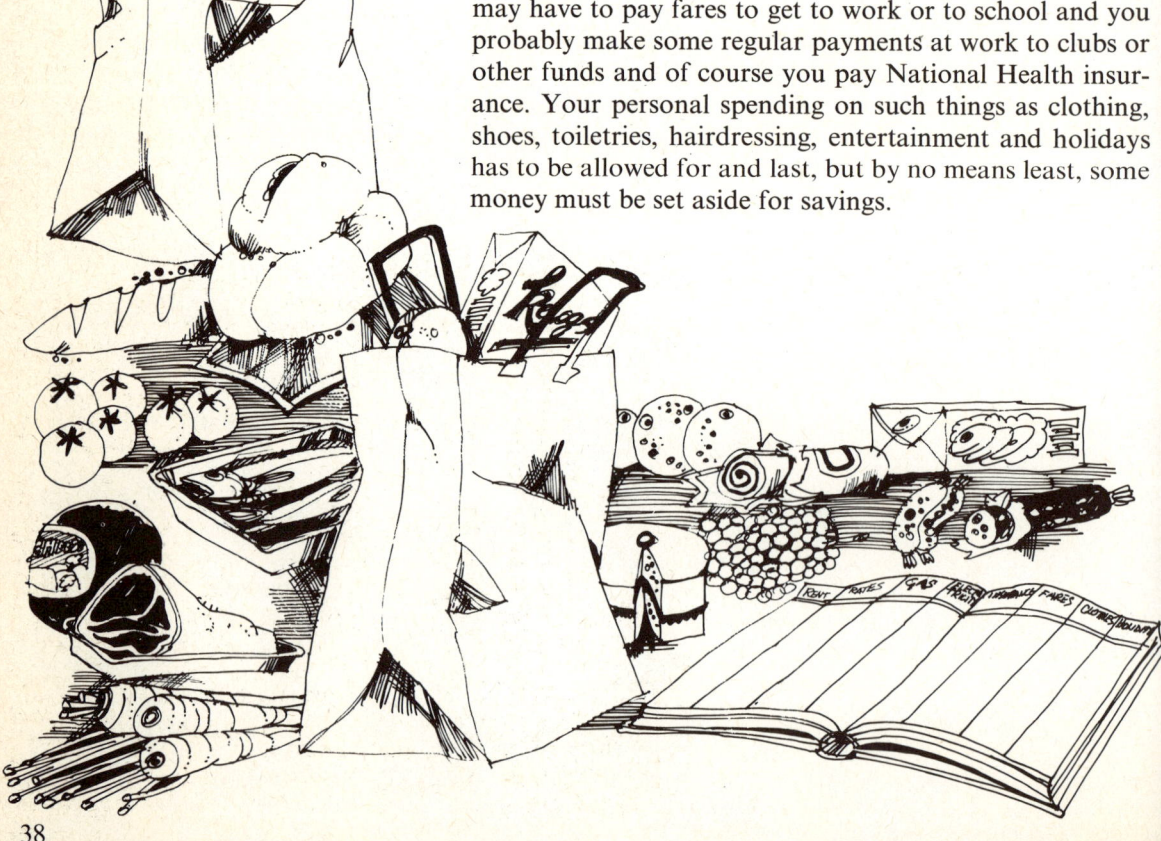

With so many things for which money must be allowed it is absolutely necessary to plan carefully, that is to make a budget and in this budget to allow enough money for adequate food. Each household must decide how to apportion the money and where economies can be made but economies in buying food must never allow the family's diet to be inadequate for their nutritional needs.

You will, of course, want to get the best value possible for your money and at the same time to do the shopping as quickly and conveniently as possible. To fulfil both these aims there are several things to decide.

WHERE TO SHOP

Although they may not all be near your home there are several types of shops to choose from and it is worth while to consider their relative advantages or disadvantages.

First consider the *local shop*, which may be a more or less general store and extra useful if it is also a post office; you can list some of its attractions and uses but economically it may not have space to store large amounts of goods and therefore may have to pay comparatively high wholesale prices, which are naturally passed on to the customers. There are also shops dealing in one type of food such as the

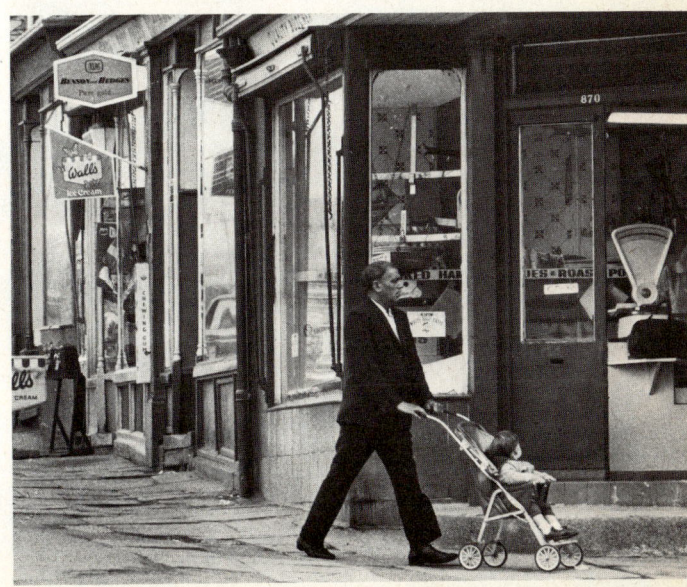

butcher, greengrocer or baker. In these, although you can generally only buy one kind of food you can sometimes get advice about your choice; many butchers will tell you which meat is of the best value and even the best way to cook it. They are all experts in their own trade but they may each cater for one particular kind of customer and the quality and price of their goods may vary according to the demands of their own clientele.

To buy different kinds of food in one shop you can go to *self-service shops* or *supermarkets*: the difference between these is their size and their range of goods. A *self-service shop* may not be very big (in fact many are a little cramped) and its stock may not include the whole range of foodstuffs. A *supermarket* is much larger, there is plenty of space to move around and usually every type of food is stocked though fish is usually only of the frozen kind. Both these types of shop reduce the cost of their wages bill by having no counter-hands (though, if you stop to think, a great deal of work is needed to stock the shelves and price every item) and they can usually buy in large quantities, particularly if they belong to a chain of stores. Prices in these shops may be less than in the individual shops but they also vary from store to store. The large supermarkets can usually afford to

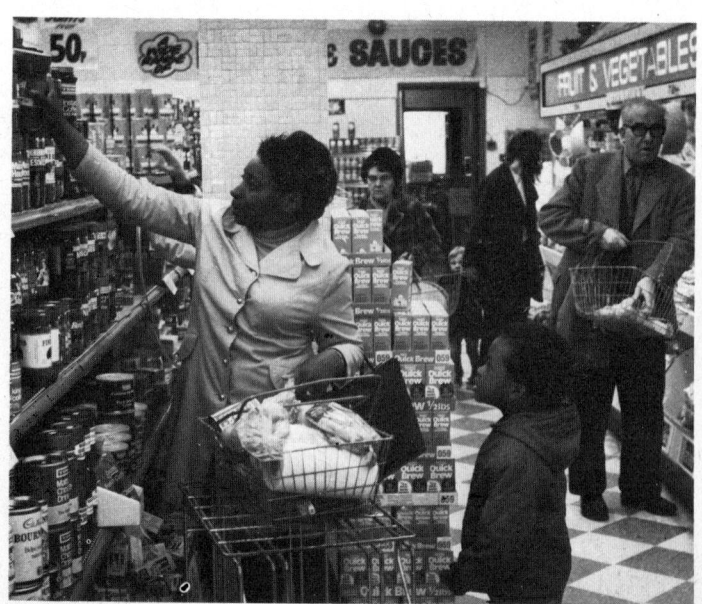

make a comparatively small profit on their very large volume of sales and can offer the lowest prices.

You can no doubt think of advantages and disadvantages of self-service and supermarket shopping but remember, the store is out to make money and relies on the fact that shoppers may be tempted by the wide and varied array of goodies to buy things they had not thought of and perhaps do not really need: they call this *impulse buying*. As a keen shopper out for good value, you need to develop a certain amount of *sales resistance* and to refuse to have your own judgment clouded by subtle advertising. Notice, next time you are in a supermarket, which items are arranged close to the check-out desks.

The difficulties, for the shopper, in deciding on the best value for money are many. For example, goods are not always packed in equal amounts; the weight may not be clearly printed on the pack; the stores 'own brands', though often cheap, may not be of the quality she wants; 'special offers' or 'special reductions' may be reduced from a price higher than that in another store and it takes time, energy and quick mental arithmetic to 'shop around' comparing prices from shop to shop.

Another way to shop is in *street markets* or at *street stalls*. The stallholder has not many overheads (but he does pay

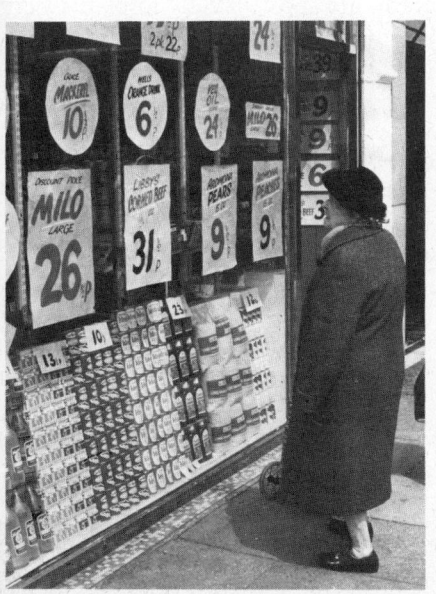
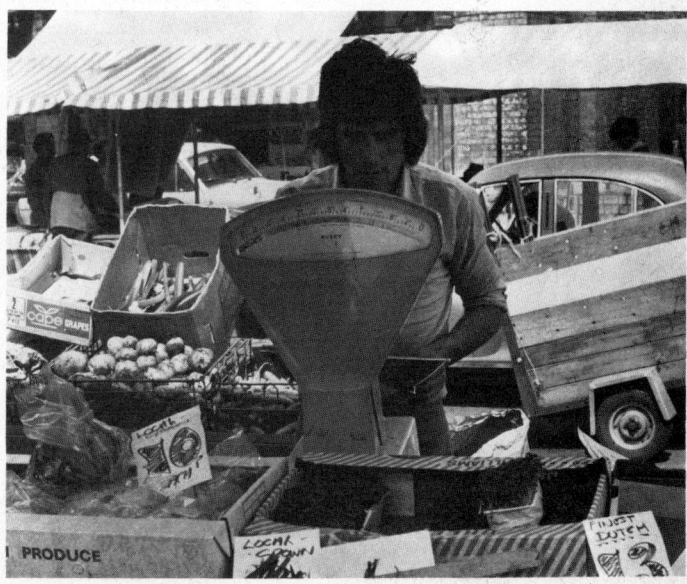

market dues and provide his own transport). He can probably afford to charge less for his goods than do shops, also, as he usually has little or no room to store them, his vegetables and fruit are usually fresh. In buying from a market stall notice the quality of the wares displayed because some small traders only buy the cheapest goods at the wholesale market and of course aim to sell even damaged items to any unwary customer, though most stallholders give very good value.

In deciding at which shop to get the best value for money it may be necessary to consider the cost of transport. If the shops offering the lowest prices are some way away from your home you will need to decide if the bus or train return fare is less than the amount you save on your purchases. If it is more you may save time and energy shopping nearer home, except for a special expedition now and then.

CLEAN SHOPS

As well as watching prices it is important to notice how clean are the shops which sell perishable foods. This is because many 'tummy upsets', diarrhoea and sickness, are directly caused by bacteria in food. These illnesses, if severe, are really dangerous and only sensible food hygiene can guard against them. The bacteria are most usually implanted on food by human beings—by dirty hands, by droplets from coughs or sneezes or by dirty clothes or aprons; less often nowadays by flies, rats and mice, but often by domestic pets.

The conditions under which bacteria can multiply to dangerous levels are warmth and moisture.

The foods on which bacteria are most likely to multiply dangerously are:

meat
milk and cream
fish
sweetened synthetic or real cream on cakes, pastries and desserts
all cooked mixtures especially meat, meat pies and milk mixtures
sometimes damaged fruit and vegetables
duck eggs

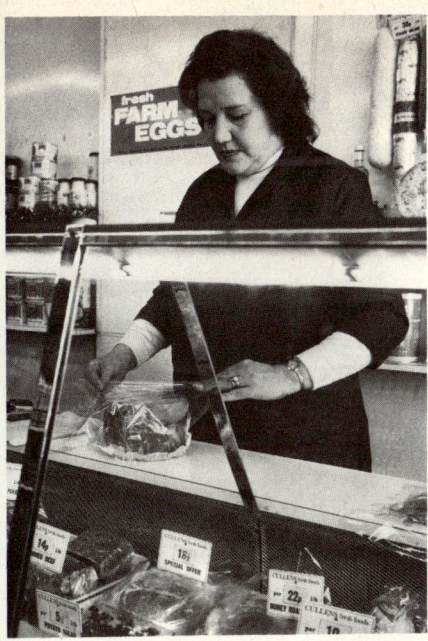

To shop safely

Choose only shops where perishable foods are kept cool and covered and/or screened by glass from customers and above all where the sale of food is quick and where no stale food is offered. The move towards date-stamping all packeted perishable foods is an excellent idea. The shop itself must be spotlessly clean, and so, of course, must the assistants be, with clean aprons and clean hands; even so they should never handle unwrapped foods, especially cooked meat, but should lift the food with tongs or covered with grease-proof paper.

Even a deep freeze cabinet can provide hazards. Packets stored above the *load-line* do not always remain frozen and once thawed frozen food goes bad more quickly than fresh food; if refrozen it will be even worse contaminated.

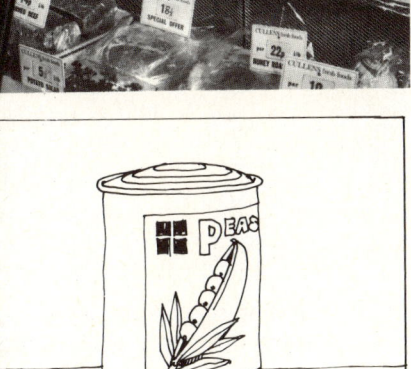

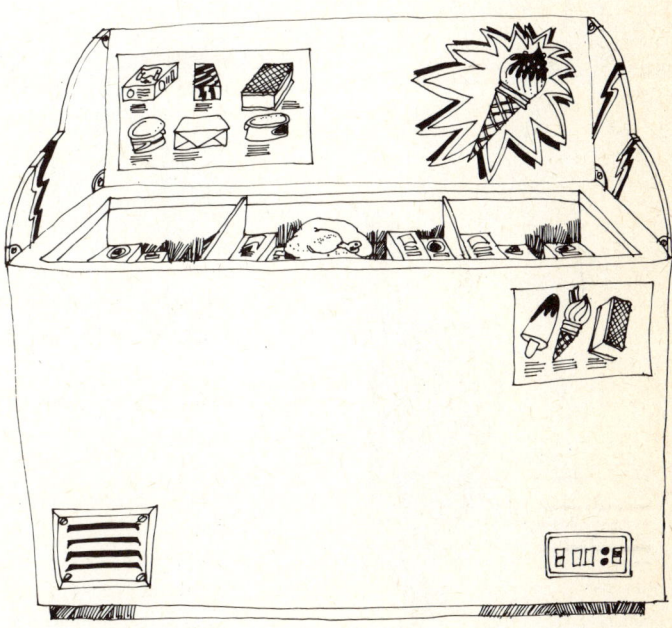

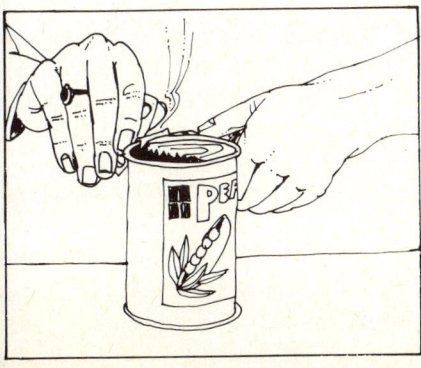

Canned foods are normally perfectly safe, but if the can has a bulge this will probably have been formed by a gas produced by bacteria inside the can and the contents will be definitely poisonous.

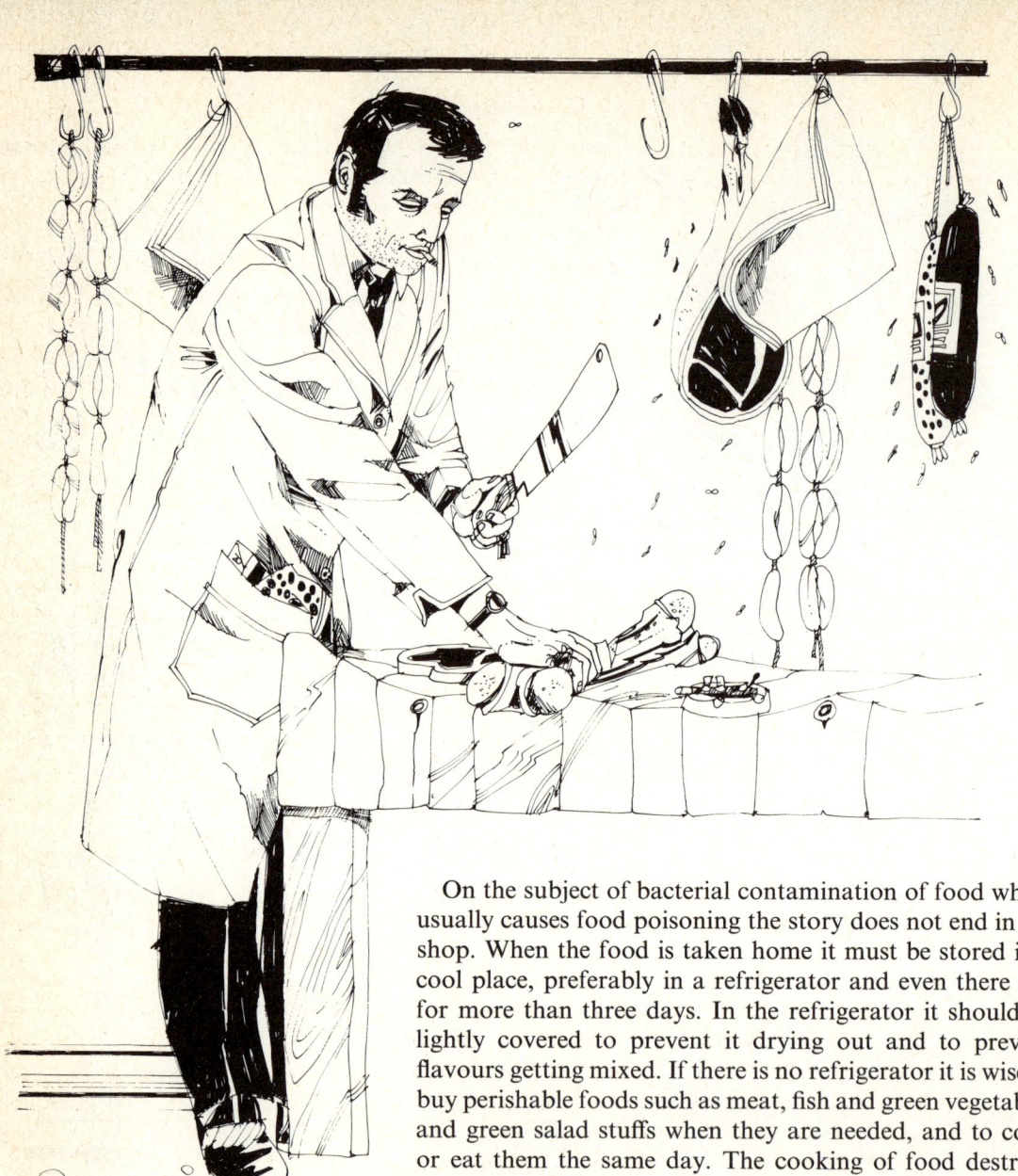

On the subject of bacterial contamination of food which usually causes food poisoning the story does not end in the shop. When the food is taken home it must be stored in a cool place, preferably in a refrigerator and even there not for more than three days. In the refrigerator it should be lightly covered to prevent it drying out and to prevent flavours getting mixed. If there is no refrigerator it is wise to buy perishable foods such as meat, fish and green vegetables and green salad stuffs when they are needed, and to cook or eat them the same day. The cooking of food destroys bacteria provided it is thoroughly cooked. Partial cooking, or slow reheating so that the inside of the food is only warm for some time will allow bacteria to multiply.

The safest rule is to cook only enough for the family's needs and to serve it while hot: if any is left over or if the dish is to be used cold, cool it quickly and keep it cold and covered.

How often you shop for your household must depend on the space you have for storing food and how suitable it is. For dry goods, dry airy cupboards are needed and for perishable foods a really cold place. If there is not much space then shopping must be done a little at a time and often, but this is usually costly as larger packs are nearly always much more economical than small ones. The cheapest way to buy non-perishable foods is by 'bulk-buying' at, for example, a 'cash and carry' shop but this is obviously ridiculous unless you have plenty of suitable storage space or can share the purchases with friends. In any case when there is plenty of any good thing you may tend to use it extravagantly and many, even dry, groceries deteriorate in a few weeks or months.

In normal household storage space, dry groceries such as tea, sugar, flour, spices and canned foods will keep well for several months, but some foods soon deteriorate. Some cereals, such as rice or semolina, may develop tiny beetles or weevil; chocolate and coffee will lose flavour and dried fruits may become too dry or, in damp weather, ferment and fats and oils may go rancid. These are rare occurrences but it is not wise to store these foods for more than a few weeks.

However frequently or infrequently you shop, before you set out make a list so that you do not forget anything; decide how much you can spend and take a large enough bag or basket to hold everything.

THE SHOPPING LIST

Turning back to chapter 1 we can use the food groups as a framework for our shopping list for the week's food.

In *Group I*, on which of the building foods can we economise? Certainly not on milk because, as we know, each member of the family should have at least half a pint daily and at least one pint if he or she is still growing. We can choose between several grades of milk for which the price is fixed; the dearer grades simply have more cream, not more protein, or they have been homogenised. Eggs, being most valuable builders, at a fixed price are very good value in protein for money; the choice here is between sizes (standard eggs are large enough for most needs) and colour of shell. Brown shelled eggs are not nutritionally any different

45

from white ones and are certainly not worth the higher price that some shops charge for them.

The price story for meat is different. The expensive and popular cuts such as fillet steaks may be nearly four times as costly as beef for stewing; similarly with mutton, lamb and pork, some cuts are always much cheaper than the prime ones. Imported meat is usually cheaper than the home-fed and home-killed varieties, and the relative prices of meat from different animals will vary from time to time. Your butcher will advise you on the best value on any one day.

In buying meat and, when we come to it, fish, it is wise to keep an open mind when making your list so that you buy the kind that is the best value on that day.

The differences in price between different cuts of meat depend usually on the relative tenderness and the relative amount of waste. The cheaper cuts that have little waste will certainly need careful cooking to make them as tender as the expensive ones, but their protein value is just as high and even taking into account a high proportion of bone, some cheap cuts such as breast or neck of lamb compare favourably as to price and food value with the prime cuts. These cheaper cuts can be made into delicious casseroles, pies and meat puddings and the tasty dishes that can be made with minced meat are numberless. If we are catering economically, grilling, frying or roasting prime meat must be special treats for special occasions. Chicken nowadays is a reasonably economical form of meat whether for roasting or in joints for grilling, frying or using in a casserole.

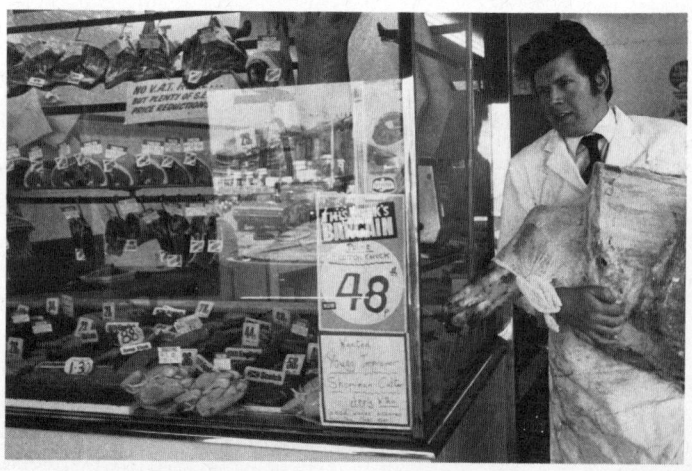

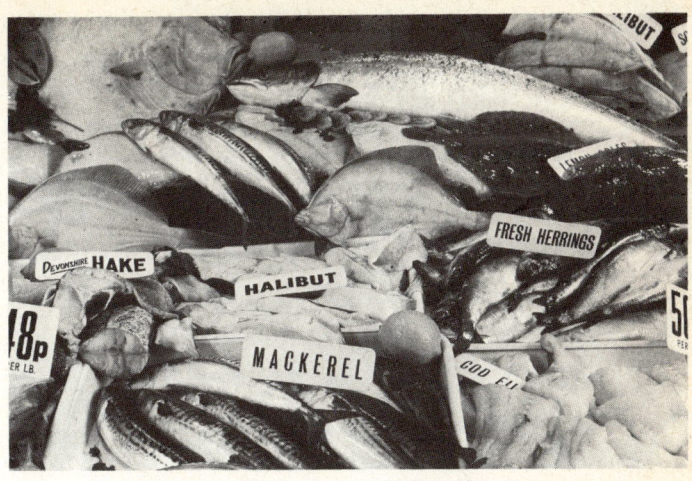

As well as choosing cheaper cuts, meat can often be made to go further by stuffing it or adding baked beans, or soaked haricot beans or other pulses to a casserole or, like the French, including sausages in the recipe.

Fish, also in group I, is another building food on which it is easy to economise as the food value of all white fish is very much the same but the prices differ widely. In the inexpensive group are rock-fish or huss, and saithe, pollack, coley or coal fish, which are cheaper than cod or fresh haddock and can be just as appetising if cooked and served with equal care. Herrings and mackerel are not only cheap but delicious to eat and especially valuable nutritionally because of the vitamins A and D which they contain. Some canned fish, usually the valuable kinds listed also in Group V, are good value for money. In buying fresh fish the price for whole fish, especially the flat kinds, is deceptive as you may be paying for fifty per cent or more of bone and head. If you do buy whole fish remember the fishmonger will usually scale, skin or fillet it and even bone herrings just for the asking, and he does this more skilfully and more quickly than you can yourself.

While considering group I it is worth noting that the building foods on which vegetarians rely are (with the exception of some nuts) very much cheaper than meat or fish and can be most appetising, as the popularity of baked beans shows. Cheese is always an economical building food compared with meat or fish because it contains much more

47

concentrated protein as well as a relatively high proportion of calcium for a much lower price—unless you buy the luxury varieties. See p. 117 for meat substitutes.

In group II we can really put our knowledge of food values to good use in spending our money wisely. The prices of fruit and vegetables, on which we rely for vitamin C, for much of the vitamin B complex and for minerals, vary enormously between the different kinds and according to the season. For vitamin C thin-skinned small oranges generally give the best value; one of them will usually supply enough vitamin for one day and is usually cheaper than half a grapefruit or a couple of ounces of soft summer fruit. Among green leaf plants watercress has nearly six times as much vitamin C as lettuce, weight for weight, and is usually much cheaper. Cabbage and brussel sprouts are also very much better value than lettuce, the more so because we usually eat more of them by weight than we do of lettuce; a quarter of a pound of cabbage is a reasonable helping but a quarter of a pound is an awful lot of lettuce. There is a catch here, however, because cabbage and sprouts are usually cooked and unless this is carefully done at least half the vitamins and mineral salts are lost. However, both are very good raw in salad, as also are raw cauliflower and raw carrot, and these together with watercress make very good substitutes for the conventional and usually costly lettuce, tomato and cucumber.

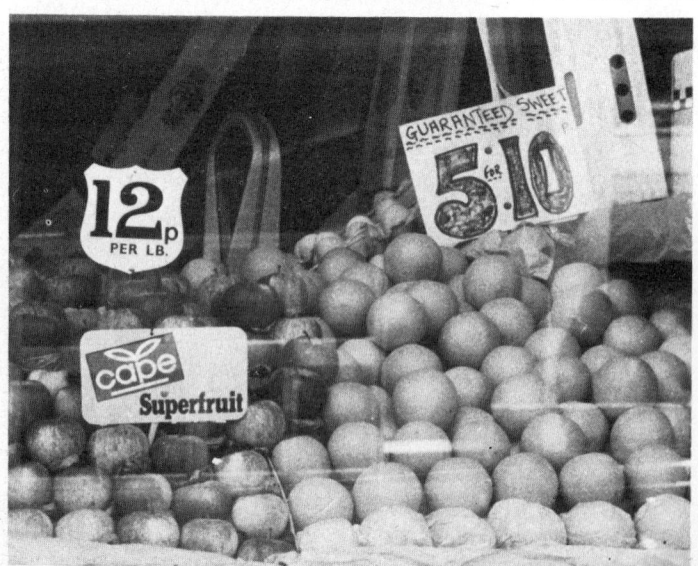

In *Group III* margarine is a very good substitute for butter because as well as being much cheaper in this country it must by law contain a good proportion of both vitamins A and D, both of which are variable in butter. Some vegetable oils are relatively cheap and can substitute for costly olive oil for salads and for other fats for frying.

In *Group IV* the simpler, more homely items such as bread, potatoes, rice and oatmeal are all comparatively cheap and are all useful for the small amounts of protein, minerals and vitamins which they contain as well as the absence of the worst fattening, tooth-destroying food in this group—sugar. It is in this group of fuel foods that money can most easily be saved. Such goodies as cakes, sweet biscuits, sweetened breakfast cereals and sweets are all comparatively expensive, and much as we may like them they are all enemies of good teeth and good figures.

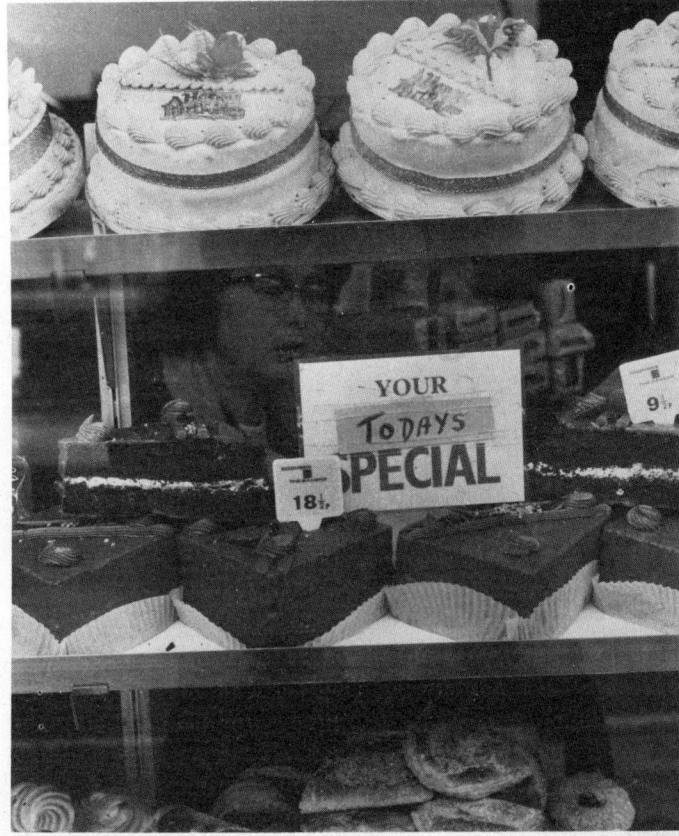

Things to do

Shop around

1. Make a shopping list for a few items that you might need for family meals. Then, looking in various shops, see if you can find much difference in prices of each article. Window shop as far as possible—in most shops you will have to buy something small otherwise you may find yourself unwelcome.
2. Compare the prices of different kinds of fish and of different cuts of meat.
3. Can you find any differences in the prices of vegetables or fruit between stalls and shops?
4. Make a note of the fluctuation of prices of fish, meat and vegetables and fruit over several weeks and account for them if you can.

Further reading

CONSUMER COUNCIL. *About Shopping,* 1972.
CONSUMER COUNCIL. *About Buying Food and Drink,* 1972.
HUGGET, R. *Shops,* Batsford, 1969.
MABEY, RICHARD. *Food,* Penguin Education, Connexions, 1972.
BRITISH FARM PRODUCE COUNCIL. Pamphlets: Choosing for Quality—Green Vegetables; British Cheeses; Meat.

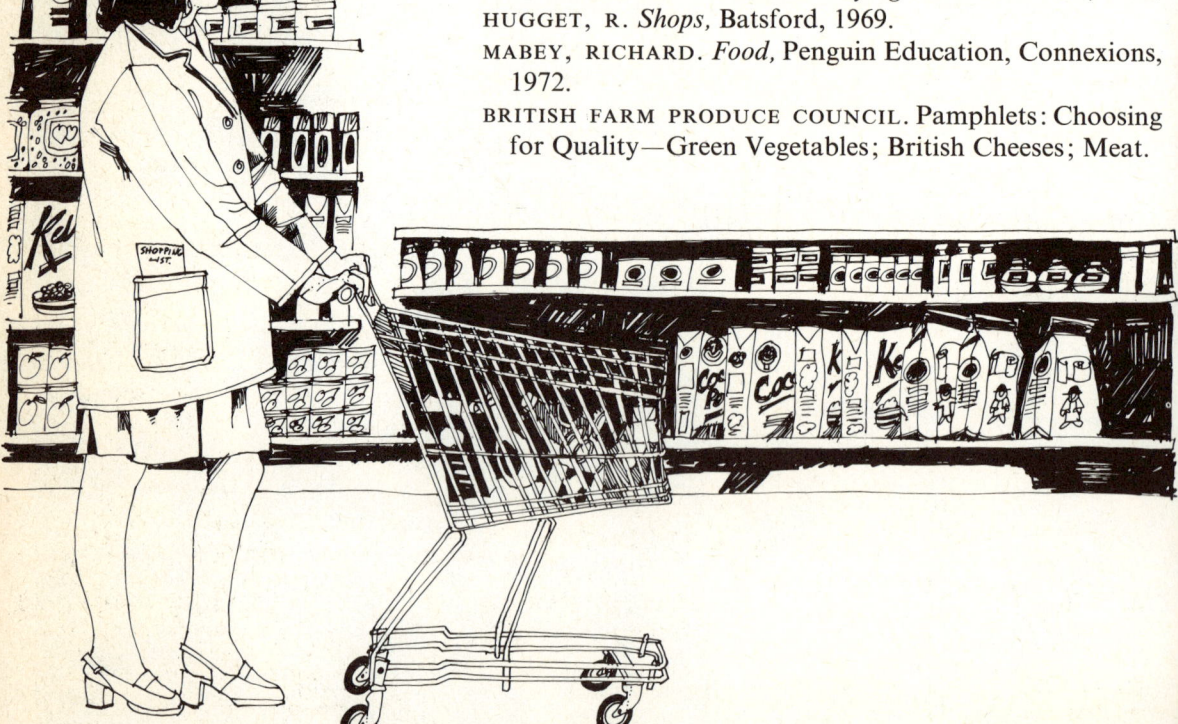

4 No Time to Cook

There are many families in which the chief housekeeper and cook, usually of course mother, also goes out to work and has only a short time to get together a meal for her family in the evening. The evening meal varies in importance according to the midday meals that the family have had. As you probably worked out from chapter 2, snack midday meals vary widely in nutritive value and of course, good as they may be, school meals that are not eaten do no one any good. So to be well fed, the family may have to rely on a good breakfast and a good evening meal—tea, supper or dinner—whatever it is called.

PLANNING AND EQUIPMENT

With little time to cook how does the meal provider manage? There are many ways, some of them very expensive. First she may have equipment designed to save time, for example a pressure cooker reduces to a third or a quarter the cooking time for most foods, and an automatically timed oven can be set so that while the cook is out of the house the meal is cooked and is ready and hot when she comes home.

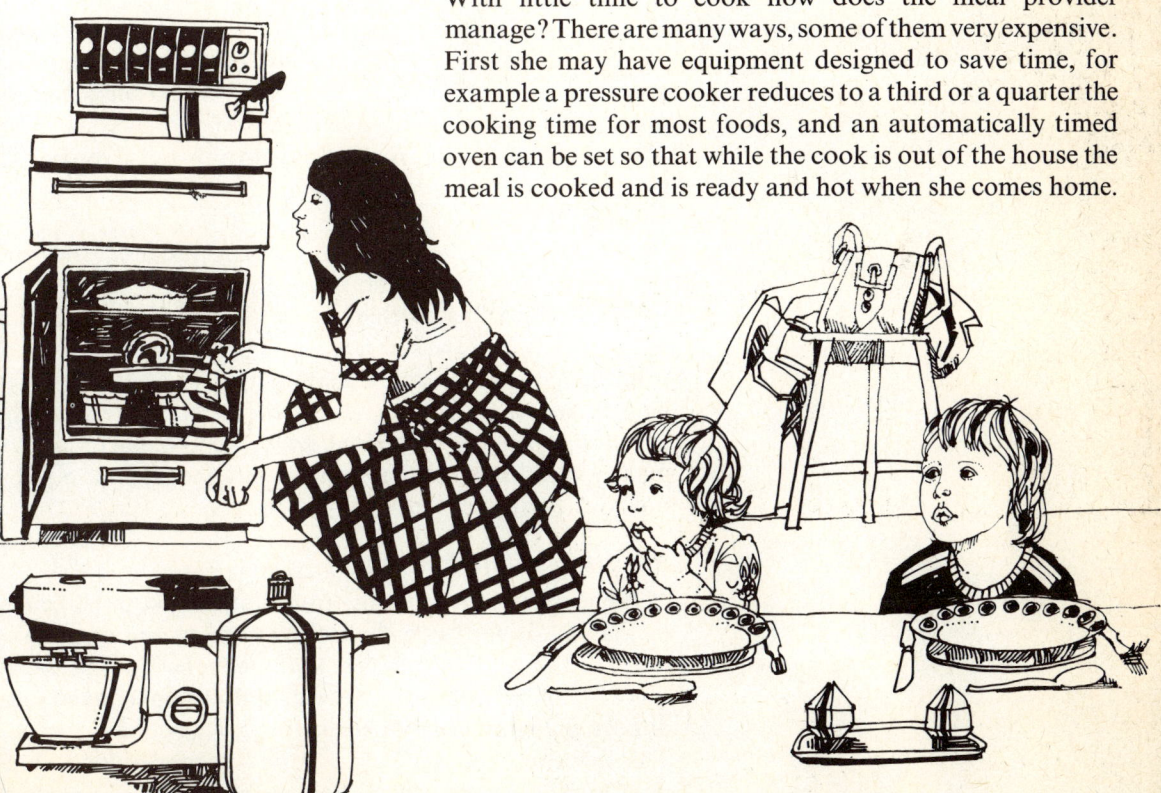

Both these devices need some planning; the pressure cooker particularly must be used strictly according to the rules issued with it, and for a meal to be cooked successfully in an automatically timed oven all the dishes should need approximately the same time and oven-heat. Other costly devices for saving time are electric mixers, blenders or whisks and food freezers.

CONVENIENCE FOODS

The very many prepared or packaged foods, clumsily called 'convenience foods', are specially intended for cooks with little time. They vary from complete meals and packet mixes for cakes, puddings, soups or sauces to single food items. They may be canned (sometimes with two compartments in the can), dehydrated (dried) and sealed in a packet or foil container, or deep frozen and sold from the shop's freezer cabinet. The range of convenience foods is far too wide to list here; some of them are excellent, for example frozen packs of fish and some vegetables; some do not provide much nutritive value for money; some are quite complicated to prepare; but all of them save time though many are more expensive than similar foods bought fresh and unprepared.

Canned foods

These are cooked during the canning process; they are sealed in cans while hot, air being drawn out before sealing, and the cans are then further heated to sterilise them. Canned foods are some of the safest we can buy as they are kept free from bacteria while they remain sealed. A faulty seal may be detected at once as either the contents ooze out or the can develops a bulge caused by poisonous bacteria producing a gas. In either case do not buy the can but point it out to the shopkeeper.

Modern dehydrated foods

These are different from the traditional dried peas, beans, lentils and dried fruits which need soaking and sometimes long cooking. The modern kinds can be cooked fairly quickly, often without soaking and, when cooked, are almost indistinguishable from the fresh cooked original. This is because modern dehydration is carried out in a short time by passing the vegetables and fruits over a current of

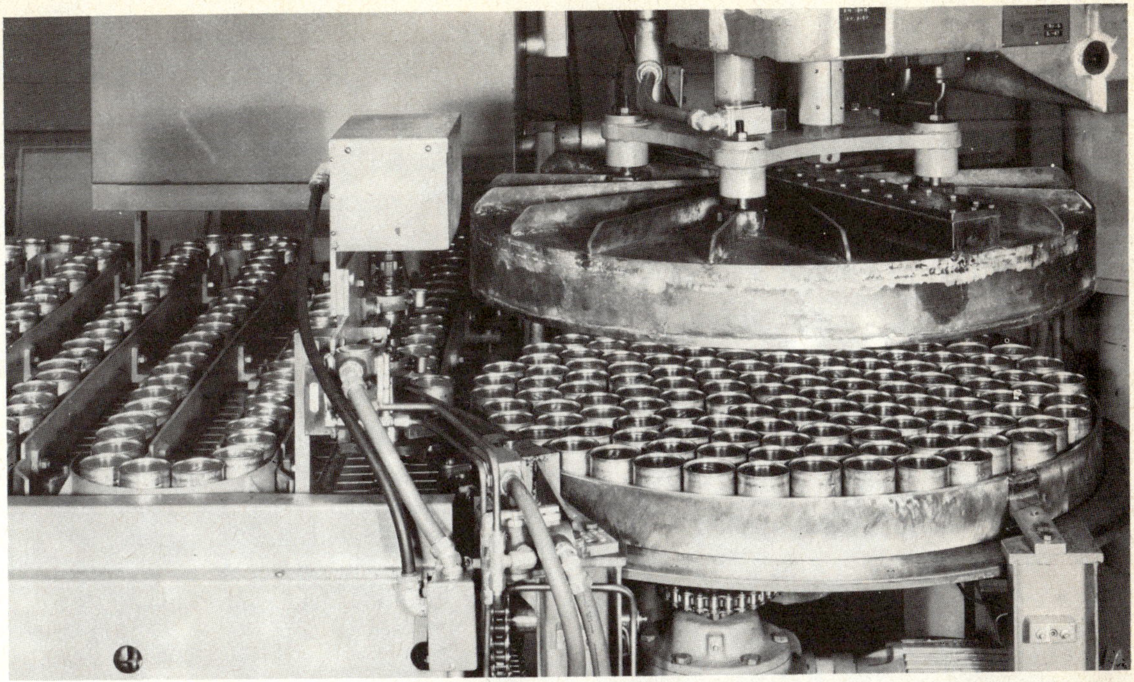

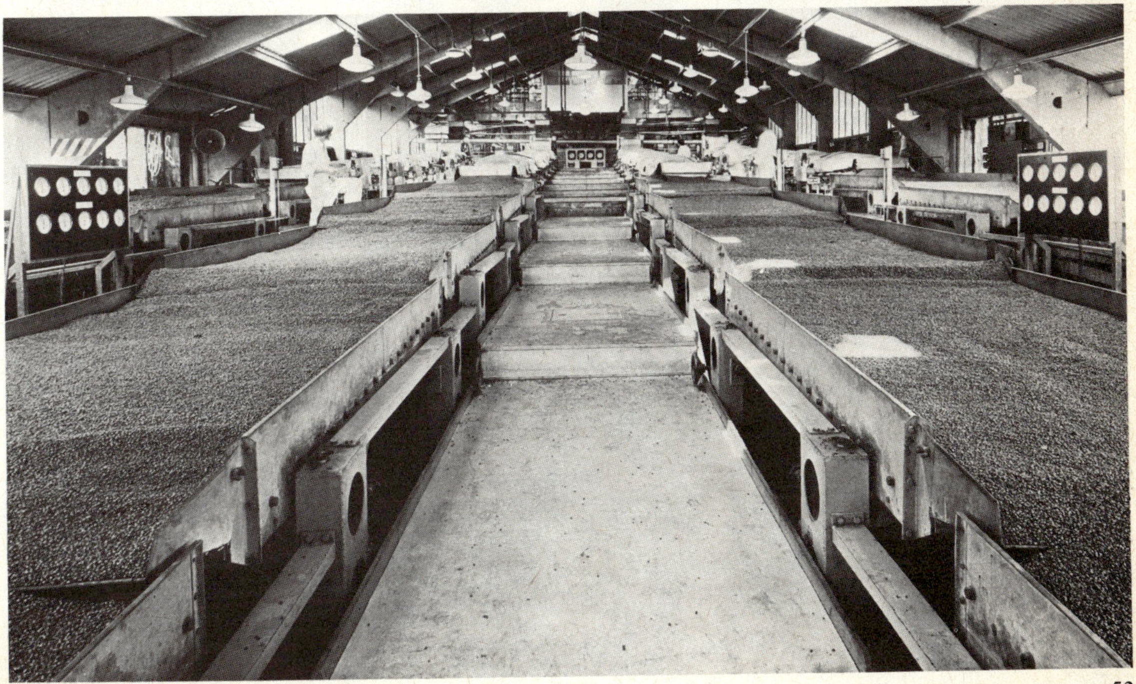

hot air. This method does not destroy so many of the water soluble vitamins as did the older, slower method.

Another method of dehydration is 'A.F.D.', that is accelerated freeze drying by which, just as the name tells us, the food is first quick frozen and then dried quickly under reduced air pressure. This process renders the food porous and easy to restore to its original moist state. It is not much used for the retail market but for the catering trade many items of fish, meat and vegetables are so treated as are some of the pieces of meat or fish in packs of dried curry and other made up dishes.

Deep frozen foods

These are frozen at temperatures as low as $-30°C$ and stored at $-18°C$; they may or may not need thawing before use (instructions on the pack tell you which), and unless they are used at once must be stored in the freezing compartment of a refrigerator or in a home freezer. In shops they must be stored below the load line in a freezer cabinet.

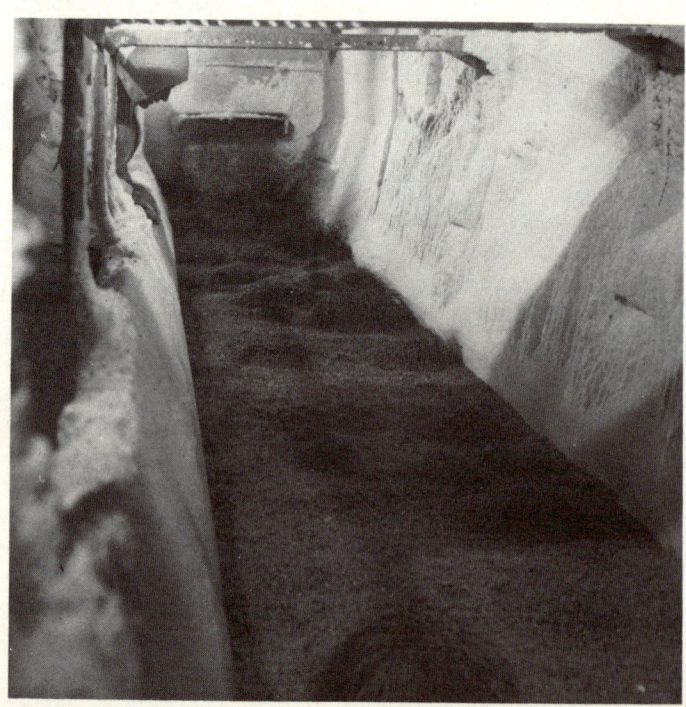

Using convenience foods

Convenience foods are not the whole answer to everyone who has little time to cook. For one thing many of them turn out to be a costly way of buying the nutrients they contain, and, for another, many people, in spite of limited time, enjoy cooking. For such people it is sensible to combine prepared food items with fresh foods and to use their own skill and inventiveness to work out quick ways of making whole dishes and meals.

For anyone really sold on convenience foods it is worth while to compare the price and, as far as possible, the nutritive value of any whole prepared dish with its equivalent made with fresh ingredients, then to decide whether the saving in time outweighs any difference in cost and food value.

One point to notice about savoury prepared foods such as soups, sauce-mixes and made up meat dishes is that if they all tend to taste very much alike it is because a harmless ingredient, made from wheat-germ and called mono-sodium-glutamate, is added to many such mixtures. It has a taste rather like both mushroom and chicken and it can persuade your palate that you really are eating far more of these foods than is the case.

PLANNING FOR QUICK COOKING

When planning the meals if there is little time to cook them it is obvious that the foods chosen must be those that can be cooked in the time available.

For the main, building course of a meal, that is *food from Group I* it is unfortunate that meat that can be cooked quickly is also the most expensive, for example steak for frying or grilling and chops cost more than cuts for stewing or slow roasting. However, cuts of meat that can be cooked in very little time without excessive cost are many. They include chicken joints, New Zealand lamb chops, spare-rib pork chops, minced beef, sausages, some cuts of bacon and imported liver. Roast joints and casseroles will probably be cooked only at a weekend, but most casseroles can be cooked one evening, without constant watching and reheated the next evening. In a pressure cooker tough meat can be made tender in thirty minutes' cooking time—three-quarters of an hour from start to serving time.

All kinds of fish can be cooked in a short time. The cheaper ones, such as coley or saithe, rock fish and herrings, can be cooked just as quickly as the more expensive kinds and their nutritive value is often higher.

There are many quick dishes that can be made with eggs, and cheese, and pasta or rice can be most appetisingly mixed with cooked meat, bacon, cheese or fish.

For the vegetable part of the meal (*Group II*) obviously salads save cooking time but unless they are fairly simple, say one or two vegetables only, they take some time to prepare and mix. Remember that lettuce is only cheap in the summer and is not a good source of vitamin C. Any raw root vegetable or green vegetable can be shredded finely; beetroot is usually bought ready cooked, and celery and watercress are not expensive and only need washing.

For cooked vegetables few of the green sort take more than ten minutes to cook, cauliflower broken into sprigs, or root vegetables, sliced thin, rarely need as long as fifteen minutes, often less. For the really short cut, frozen or canned vegetables are useful, always remembering that 'processed' peas, having been first dried then canned, have little vitamin content. Some very useful prepared foods for the savoury part of a meal are dried shredded vegetables for flavouring, dried potato for 'mash' and concentrated soups used as a sauce.

The second course of a main meal need be very little trouble. It may be a cold sweet made the night before, a tart made from a batch cooked at the weekend, stewed or raw fruit, perhaps with yoghurt or ice-cream; or cheese and biscuits are usually a popular substitute for a sweet.

SPEEDING UP COOKERY

As well as using prepared foods and choosing foods that can be cooked in a short time and apart from using special equipment a good deal of time can be saved by quick methods of work. Some such time-savers are 'one stage' methods for sauces, pastry and cakes.

When there is time to make pastry, make an extra amount and either cook it as a dish for a day or so later or wrap it raw in foil or polythene and store it in a refrigerator, or just rub up the fat and flour and store the dry mix in a jar or polythene bag in the store cupboard; this mixture will keep for a week or two.

Potatoes need not always be peeled: scrub them well and pare off a strip of peel from one long side, the family can easily take off the rest at table. Extra potatoes cooked one day can be sliced and fried or mashed and reheated next day or used with dressing as potato salad.

Crushed, unsweetened wheat flakes are a quick substitute for dried crumbs for coating fried food or au gratin dishes, and most dishes requiring breadcrumbs (for example, bread sauce) can be made more quickly by soaking a slice of bread in the hot liquid and then beating it smooth.

HOME FREEZING AND REFRIGERATION

Home freezing

An expensive piece of equipment that can save the cook much time is a home freezing cabinet. It is so costly that it must be used with understanding of suitable foods to be frozen, which foods need thawing before use, and how the cabinet must be cared for. All this is explained in cheap booklets issued by most of the manufacturers. Briefly the foods usefully frozen or stored in the freezer are fish, meat, vegetables and fruit and, perhaps even more usefully,

Home freezing cabinet
Below *Upright model*
Below right *Chest model*

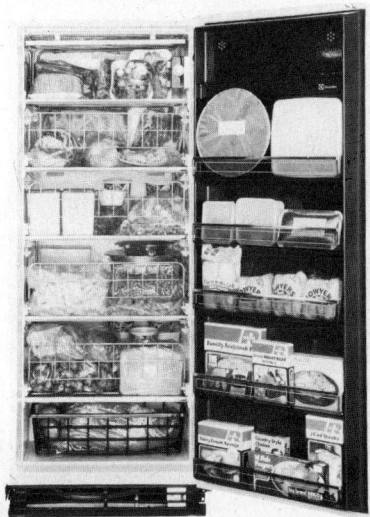
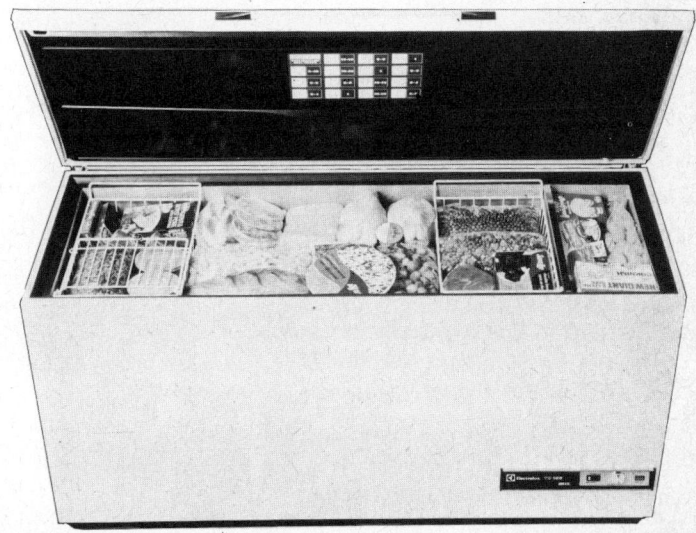

complete cooked dishes such as casseroles, curries, soups and other made up dishes and cakes. Cooked sauces and raw pastry either rolled to shape or wrapped in convenient pieces can both be stored frozen. The made dishes, of course, would be prepared when there is time to spare and at least in duplicate so that part can be used the same day and part frozen for future use.

Cooked dishes can be reheated without thawing; fish, vegetables and fruit for stewing can be cooked in the frozen state but meat, pastry, cakes and fruit to be eaten raw must be thawed before cooking or using and this thawing may take two hours or more.

Refrigerator

Not quite so costly as a home freezer, a refrigerator can save time chiefly from the shopping. A small amount of commercially frozen food can be stored in the frozen food compartment for from one to twelve weeks depending on the star rating and fresh foods, if covered with foil or polythene, can be kept in the main compartment for up to three days.

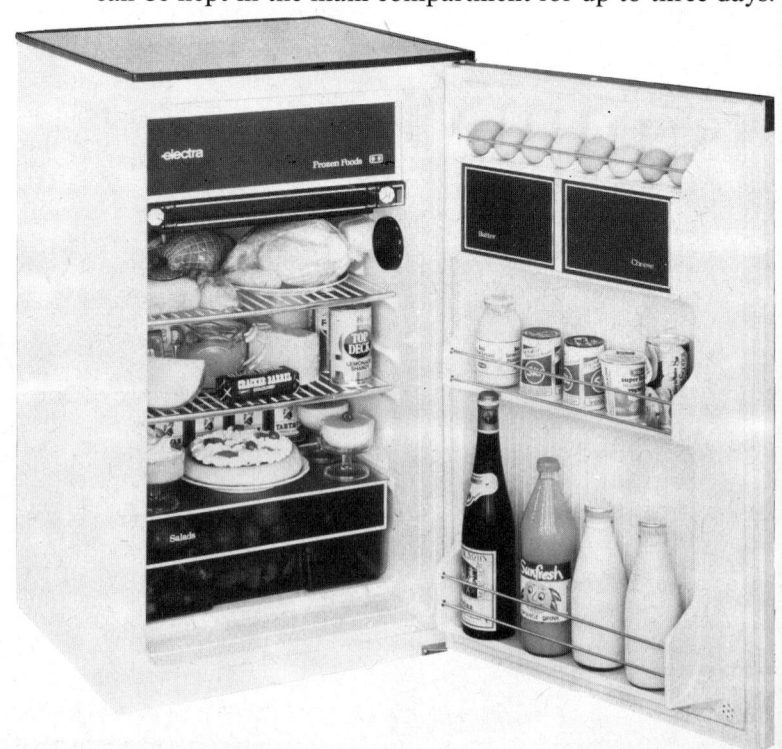

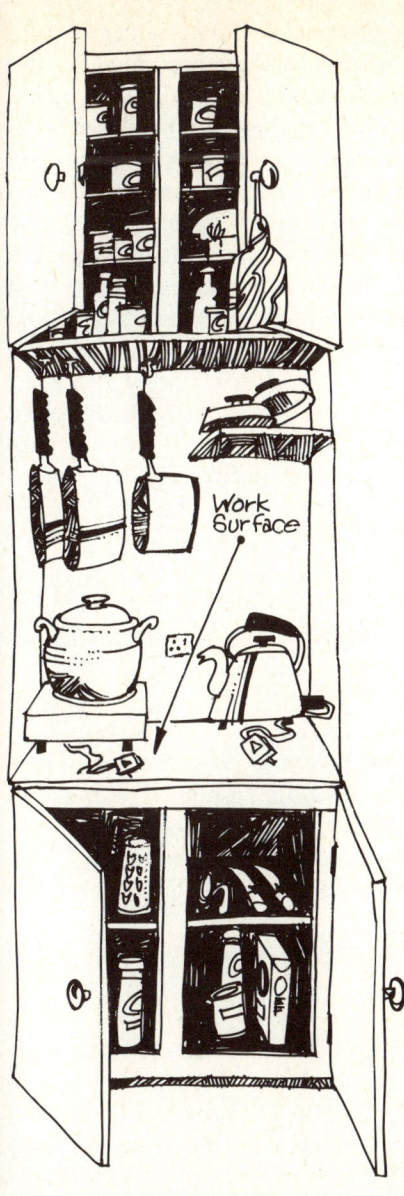

Work Surface

COOKING IN A BEDSITTER OR COOKING FOR ONE

The problems of catering for this way of life usually include not only limited money to spend but also limited space for preparing and storing food and minimal equipment for cooking it. There are many modern devices for cooking in a small space—all fairly costly. They include electric frying pans, tiny gas or electric ovens and combined grill-hot-plates. But with practice and experiment surprisingly good meals can be produced using one gas ring or electric hot-plate. Some suggested items are a strong frying pan with a lid so that it can also be used as a stew pan, a strong sauce-pan with a steamer top to fit it (which can also be used as a colander), and a smaller saucepan with a lip for pouring. If it can be afforded, some of these items can be of gaily coloured enamelled steel and will then look attractive as table-ware for entertaining. One important point is to make sure that all pans are well balanced so that they will not tip over on the gas ring. To complete the minimum kitchen outfit, a kettle, a chopping board, some knives and spoons are needed and a grater for shredding vegetables and grating cheese is also very useful.

SHOPPING FOR ONE

Because there is usually very little space and no refrigerator for storing food the greatest difficulty is buying fresh foods in sufficiently small quantities for one person's needs for one day. Some basic foods like bacon, cheese, butter, eggs and bread can be kept safely for a few days to a week and some shops are willing to sell butter by the $\frac{1}{4}$ lb (113 g). It will prob-ably be necessary to 'shop around' to find sympathetic shop-keepers who will sell small quantities of vegetables and of meat other than chops; fish can usually be bought quite easily in single portions. Green vegetables and salads can, as a rule, be stored overnight if dry and kept in a polythene bag in the dark so two days' supply can be bought at one time but meat and fish must be cooked the day they are bought as must any frozen foods where there is no refrigerator. Cooked frozen vegetables are very good in salad.

PLANNING AND COOKING FOR ONE

A meal of one main dish with vegetables followed by a sweet, if it is to be cooked on one gas ring, will need some planning and manoeuvring. It is obviously easier if one course is cold and prepared first or bought ready for table. To fit vegetables in, the steamer may be used for potatoes and other roots; cooked potatoes, tomatoes or even apple slices can be fried in the same pan with chops, gammon or bacon and eggs but of course the simplest arrangement is to have salad with hot meat. A green or a frozen vegetable takes such a short time to cook that the meat or fish can be kept warm meanwhile on a plate over the saucepan.

Some suggestions for the main, protein course of the meal, in addition to the obvious chops, bacon and eggs, liver and bacon and omelettes, include a small casserole with $\frac{1}{4}$ lb (113 g) of not too tough meat or a chicken joint with sliced dried vegetables for flavour and topped with sliced potato; a chicken joint or a chop cooked in a small can of soup or one or two eggs poached in hot canned broth or consommé. Chicken joints, either fried or grilled or a pot-roast of a very small joint or a lamb's heart are fun to try and there is a wide range of spaghetti, macaroni and rice dishes with cooked meat, liver, bacon, mince or cheese that can vary the menu.

The sweet course of a meal, as for any cook who is short of time, is easily provided if it can be cold. Worth noting is that ice cream can be kept cold for about an hour if wrapped in many layers of newspaper. A hot sweet, which is quite a rarity nowadays, needs still more manoeuvring but it can possibly be cooked (for example, a sweet omelette) while the diner(s) waits.

EATING OUT

Another way of solving the problem of meals in a bed-sitter is to eat in a café or restaurant. This, of course, is likely to be far more expensive than fending for yourself at home but occasionally it makes a good change and may give you some ideas for new dishes. It is a good plan to be a little adventurous. Select a foreign restaurant you can afford and then ask for guidance from the waiter or counterhand about dishes that are new to you. It always seems a pity to choose dishes that you can well make for yourself, at less than half the cost, such as eggs or a pasta dish, unless the latter is a real novelty to you. You will probably find that Indian,

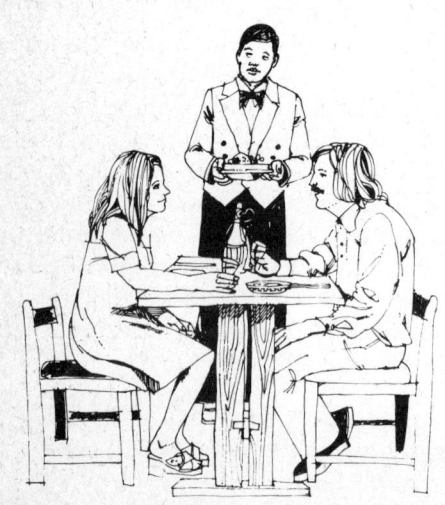

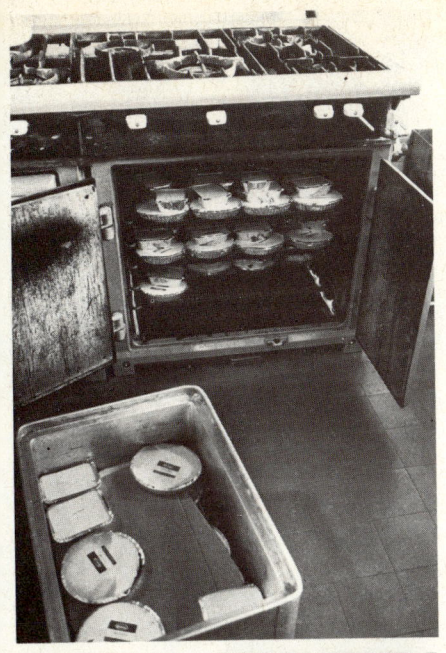

Chinese and some Greek and Italian restaurants or cafés are reasonably cheap and you can learn from their menus something of the way people eat in their countries of origin.

OLD PEOPLE ON THEIR OWN

So far we have considered cooking with limited money and limited facilities as a problem of the young single worker but it is often a much greater problem for an old person living alone, or for an old couple. Apart from the difficulties we have already considered, the shortage of money may be much more serious and as if that is not depressing enough many old people may be partially disabled by rheumatism, arthritis or some other serious disease. When beset by such troubles old people may lose confidence and interest in catering and cooking for themselves; the difficulties are so great for them that they eat the easiest foods to buy or to prepare and often have a quite inadequate diet of tea and bread and butter. Help may be available for such old people from a younger neighbour or from a home help and is particularly valuable with shopping. 'Meals on Wheels' may be available in the district and such organisations as the

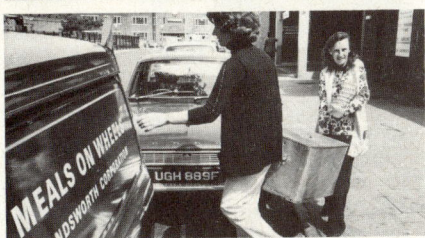

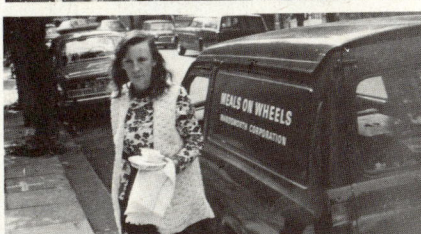

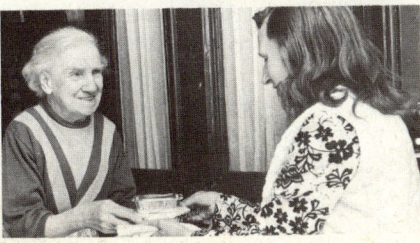

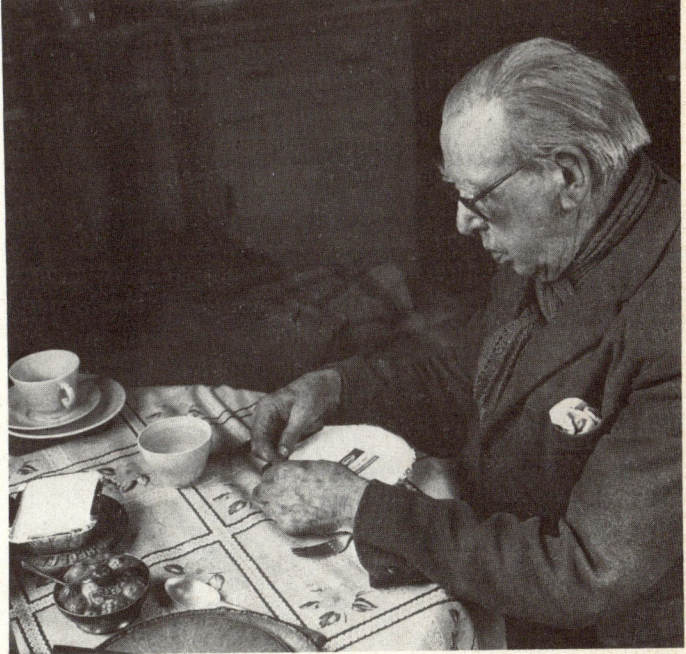

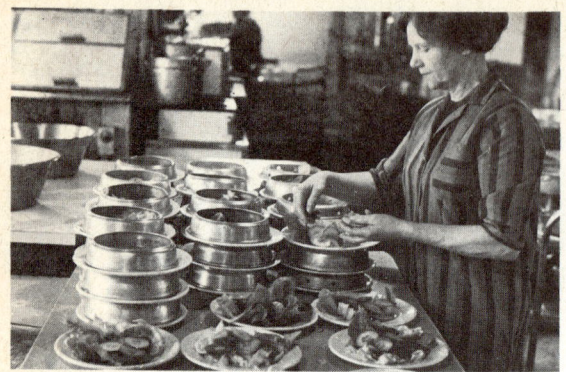 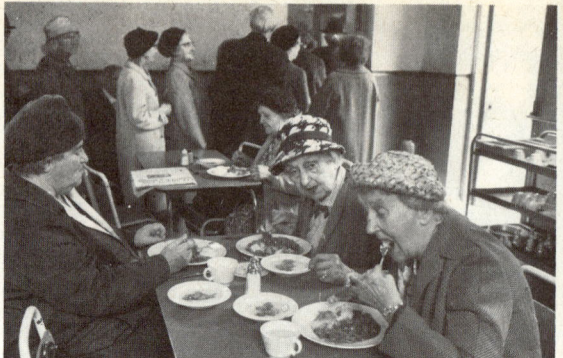

W.R.V.S. may arrange a dinner club. Meals of this kind cost very little but are only to be had on certain days in the week. For other days and for other meals shopping and cooking are still needed. As we found in chapter 2 old people do not need as much food as younger adults but the choice of their diet is, for this reason, just as important. They must have a reasonable amount of protein every day and the most easily obtained protein foods are milk, which is delivered, eggs which the milkman will usually deliver, cheese and canned meat and fish. These foods have the advantage of needing little or no cooking. Add to these bread, which most old people accept as a basic food, and they gain a little more protein along with energy food, vitamins of the B group, iron and calcium. Most of their calcium requirements they can get from milk, eggs and cheese, and for old people calcium is very important if their bones are not to become brittle.

The diet is not yet complete; it still needs fat which is probably best supplied by margarine which has a guaranteed proportion of vitamins A and D and is reasonably cheap. Also extremely necessary is some source of vitamin C. As you will remember from chapter 1 the sources of this vitamin tend to be expensive so the cheapest kinds of fruit and vegetables must be chosen. Small oranges (one a day will give a sufficient allowance) are usually cheap and so are sprouts and cabbage, which do not need much cooking. Potatoes, which often supply most of the vitamin C on a low cost diet are not a very good source except when they are new and expensive in late spring and summer.

Things to do

1. *Convenience foods price research.* Write down the price in shops of packs of frozen vegetables, fish, potato chips (*not* crisps) and note the weight or the suggested number of portions. Then, as far as you can, compare these prices with the same portions of the same foods in the fresh state. Remember to allow for waste on most fresh foods—50 per cent on some such as peas, and 25 per cent on some fish and some vegetables. Which frozen foods are good value?

2. *Working with a partner.* One of the pair buys and prepares a frozen or dehydrated or canned whole dish for which you can also find similar ingredients and a recipe and the other member prepares the dish from these. Compare the cost and the size of the portions—especially those of protein foods. Also note the time it took in each case.

3. *Labour saving equipment.* Find out the prices of electric mixers with and without all the possible attachments. Find the price of pressure cookers and the difference in price between automatic and ordinary gas and electric cookers. Find the price of home freezing cabinets.
   How much would you have to earn to be able to afford any one of these articles?

Further reading

FINN, HILDA. *No Time to Cook,* Corgi, 1967 (new edition).

WHITEHORN, KATHARINE. *Cooking in a Bedsitter,* MacGibbon & Kee, 1961; Penguin, 1970 Edition.

NATIONAL DAIRY COUNCIL PAMPHLET. *Keeping Fit in Retirement.* Not dated.

CAMERON-SMITH, MARYE. *Fresh from the Freezer,* Penguin, 1970.

CONACHER, GWEN. *Food Freezing at Home,* Electricity Council.

STORK MARGARINE CO. *The New Art of Cooking.* Also Stork Card *All in One Way.*

DAVID, LOUISE. *Easy Cooking for One or Two,* Penguin, 1972.

5 Where Food Comes From

To a towndweller food comes from shops, but if you live in the country you know that all food must come from the land; that it either grows as a plant or on a tree or it comes from an animal or bird which lives on plant food. The towndweller who keeps his eyes open when he goes into the country can see some of his food growing or walking about in a field.

IMPORTS

Originally the food for any nation was home grown, but when men travelled by land and sea they could bring back the products of other lands. At first travel was so slow that only food stuffs that would keep in good condition for

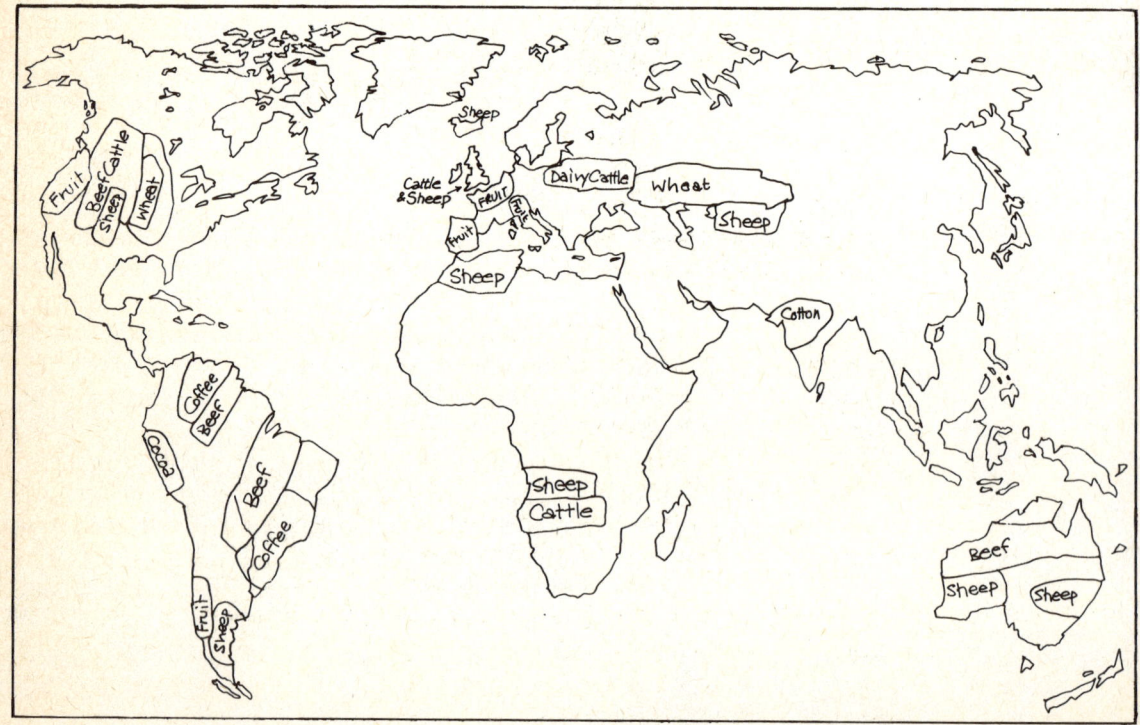

months were brought in. In Britain we imported spices from the Far East by the fifteenth century and wines from France even earlier. Later, dried fruits came from Mediterranean countries, and oranges from Spain; by the seventeenth century cocoa, coffee and tea were fashionable. When larger ships could be built, and designed to sail farther and faster, they could carry larger cargoes from more distant lands until nowadays we can import food stuffs from all over the world. Moreover, since ships have refrigerated holds and air travel has reduced long journeys to hours instead of weeks or months duration, the most perishable foods can be brought to us. The only restrictions are the cost of transport and the need for a balance of trade between the countries concerned. In other words if country A buys a great deal of anything from country B country A will expect to sell to country B products of equivalent value.

HOME PRODUCTION

In this country, in spite of our small area, we produce 60 per cent of all the food we need, and this on farms of many different sizes and on a wide variety of types of land. Geographically Britain is fortunate in the variety of her climate, soil and land contours because these are all factors which control the activities of farmers; the British farmer has chosen the livestock or the crops best suited to his land. For example, sheep and some cattle do well on hilly land that would be impossible to till for growing crops. Some types of soil are best suited to cereal crops, others to fruit or vegetables; some crops need moisture and shelter from the wind, others grow better in a drier climate. All these types of farming can be grouped as livestock-rearing for meat production, dairy farming, poultry-rearing for table birds or for eggs, arable farming for cereal crops or vegetables, fruit farming and market gardening. Because modern farming is now a highly mechanised industry and because most machines are designed to do one kind of job only, such as milking cows or harvesting grain many farms specialise in producing one kind of foodstuff. There are, however, still a number of mixed farms and farmers who rear cattle usually also grow a large proportion of the food they need, be it grass for pasturage, dried grass, silage or hay, or kale or barley.

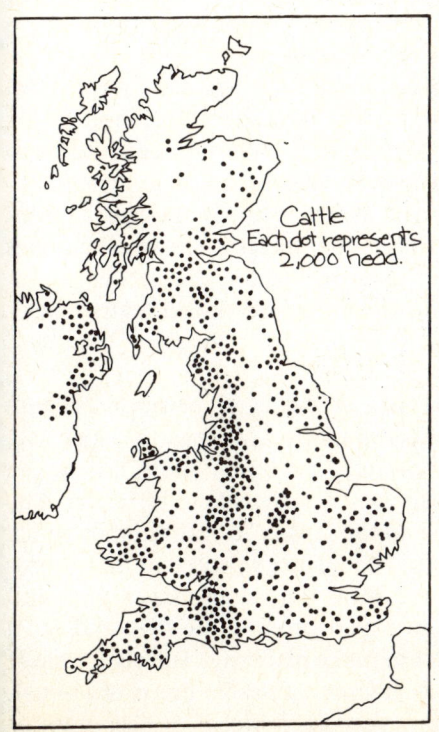

Cattle
Each dot represents 2,000 head.

All the animals now reared for meat are descended from wild ancestors which were hunted by primitive man and then, thousands of years ago, domesticated. Through the centuries modern breeds have evolved. Careful breeding and general care have developed the shape and quality of animals that are desirable and experts are constantly trying to improve the breeds still further. The health, general welfare and feeding of all farm animals is scientifically studied and the vet is a regular visitor to most stock farms. In order to ensure that the meat from all animals is free from infection they may only be killed in specially designed slaughterhouses, now called 'abattoirs', which are under strict government regulation and in which all carcases are inspected before sale.

About 75 per cent of all the meat eaten in Britain is produced in this country, the remaining 25 per cent is imported, chilled for high quality or frozen for lower grade. Beef is imported from Argentina, Australia and Yugoslavia, lamb from New Zealand and Australia (at the time of writing), with some mutton from Argentina. We do not import any fresh pork, only bacon.

Home-produced cattle, sheep and pigs are sold in local cattle markets and bought by meat traders and wholesale or retail butchers. Some of the meat is sent by meat traders to large town markets such as Smithfield in London where imported meat also arrives by refrigerated transport; from there it is distributed to regional buyers. The retail butcher has the job of cutting the meat into the size needed by his customers and to do this he must be a skilled craftsman.

Beef

Butchers have found that nowadays, perhaps because families are small and certainly because meat is expensive, their customers want relatively small joints with little waste as fat or bone. They also want all the meat to be tender. The butcher therefore looks to the farmer to rear animals which will produce such meat. The farmer's problems are to produce animals that have little fat, small bones and well developed hindquarters which provide the best and most profitable meat, and yet to make his living. To solve some of these problems he first chooses a suitable breed of animal. In Britain we have many very good breeds of beef animals,

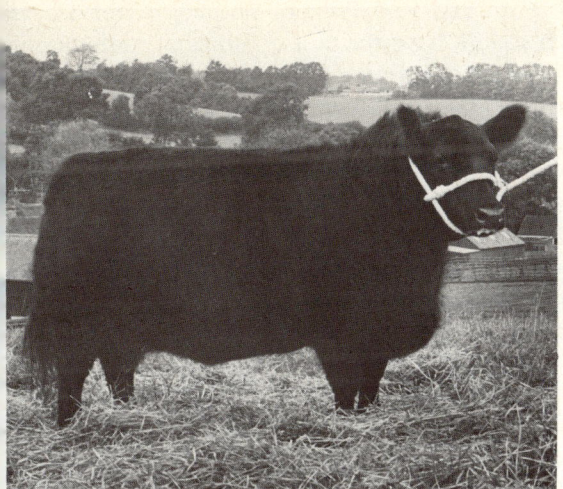

Aberdeen Angus

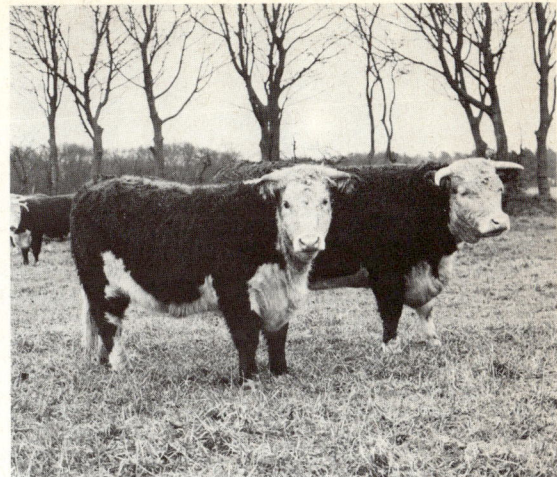

Hereford

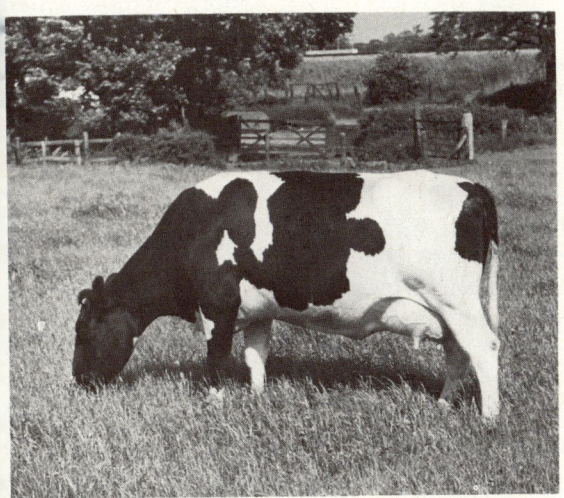

British Friesian

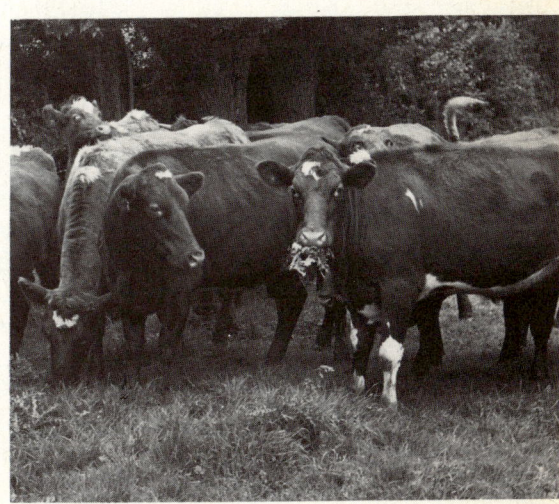

Shorthorn

many of which have been exported all over the world. Some of the famous beef breeds are, as you probably know, Aberdeen Angus, Hereford, Beef shorthorn, Lincoln Red and South Devon.

The farmer may choose to rear beef breeds or dual purpose cattle whose cows give good milk and whose male animals good beef. Some of these are British Friesian,

Dairy shorthorn and Red Poll; or he may prefer a cross breed which should have the best qualities of both parents such as Aberdeen Angus × Hereford or Aberdeen Angus × Shorthorn.

To get beef from a dairy herd, a good British beef bull or, for example, a French Charolais may be crossed with a cow from a good dairy breed to give the qualities most liked by the customer. Some farmers are using breeds from all over Europe experimentally.

Next the farmer must work out the right feeding and management of his herd so that food conversion rate is high, in other words that the animal puts on a steady increase in weight in proportion to the food he eats, and that the amount of labour needed to grow the food, to feed, water and generally look after the cattle is as low as possible and as skilled as possible.

The farmer may buy male calves at a few days old and feed them till they are ready for beef along with those reared on his farm. The animals, usually castrated males, are most carefully fed, sometimes on barley, until they are ten months to a year old, by which age their meat will be tender and their joints still small. The flavour of the meat from these young animals is not as full as the beef of some twenty years ago when two years old was the average age for slaughter and when joints were larger and had more fat.

Experiments are now being made using 'entire', untreated bulls for beef. Their growth rate is quicker and they are slaughtered before they become dangerous and difficult to manage.

Veal

Many young calves, often males from a dairy herd, are sold at a few days old for a short life before they become veal. The poorer ones who do not seem likely to 'do well' are killed as 'bobby calves' for manufacturing purposes and the rest will be most carefully fed and tended. They need skilful handling as they easily catch various diseases and for this reason veal production in Britain is on a small scale. The young animals are kept indoors in sheltered, well ventilated houses; they are not allowed much exercise which might make the veal tough and their food is specially balanced to keep their flesh white. They are ready for slaughter at eleven or twelve weeks old.

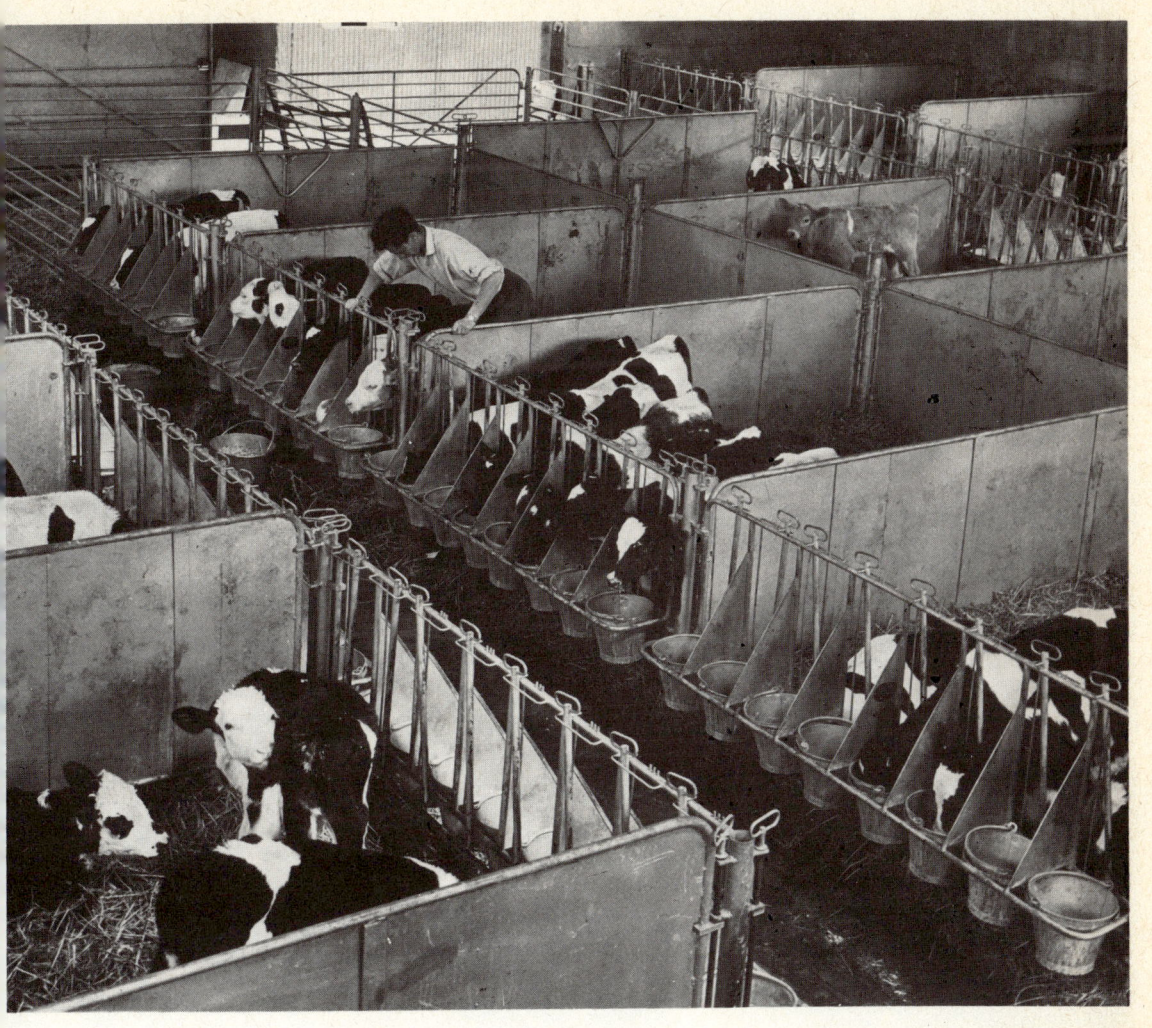

Mutton and lamb

In the past sheep were reared for their wool as much as for
meat but the present wide use of man-made fibres has
reduced the demand for wool. Perhaps this is one reason
why sheep farming has somewhat declined in this country;
another is that beef is slightly more popular with the public
than mutton. Mutton, that is meat from the fully grown
sheep, is rather out of fashion now as we seem to prefer the
more delicate flavour and the smaller joints with less fat
that lambs provide. Strong competition from New Zealand,

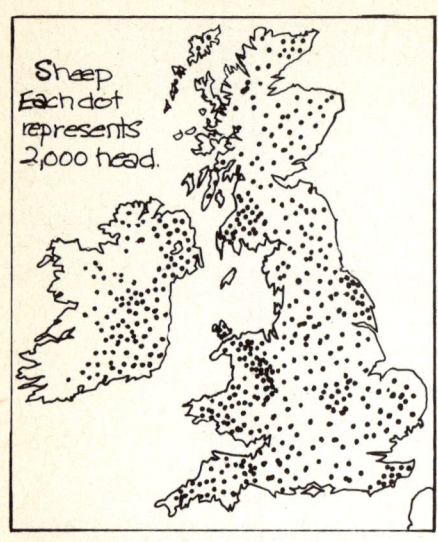

Sheep
Each dot
represents
2,000 head.

which has exported to Britain large quantities of high grade lamb at a price lower than our own home reared lamb, has discouraged the sheep farmer still further.

However, like beef cattle, there are some very good breeds of sheep in Britain. They can be divided into mountain or hill breeds which are sturdy and give well flavoured, lean meat because of the herbage on which they graze and downland or lowland breeds which give larger joints with more fat. Some of the breeds are:

Hill breeds: Welsh mountain sheep, Cheviots, Swaledales. Scotch black face.

Downland breeds: Southdown (from which New Zealand flocks of Canterbury lamb were developed), Shropshire Down, Oxford, Dorset and Hampshire Down.

Because of the popularity of lamb, modern breeding of

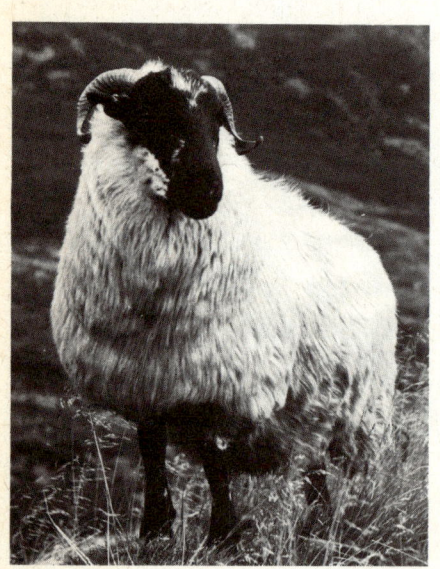

Blackface sheep

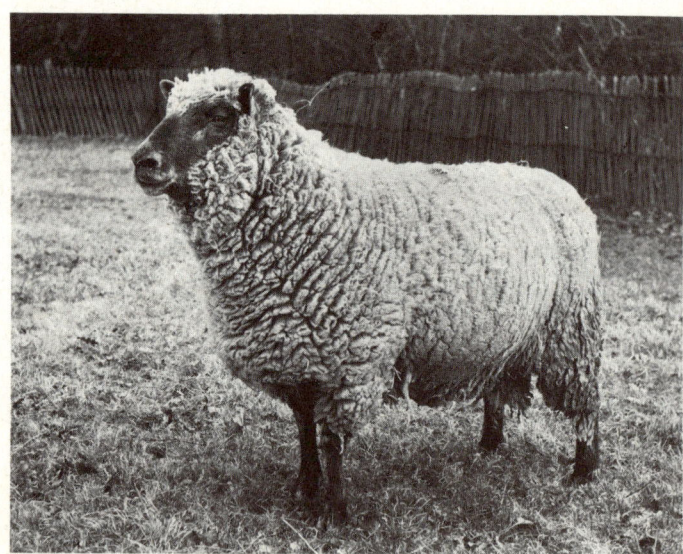

Clun ram

sheep is now aimed at developing ewes that can either produce and feed triplets, quadruplets or even quintuplets, or else can have lambs twice a year. Along with these aims modern breeding tends to develop desirable qualities which are rather like those of beef animals, that is well developed hindquarters with enough but not too much fat and a light frame. If breeding on these lines is successful we may be able to export high quality lamb to the Continent instead of importing so much.

Sheep are fed almost entirely by grazing them, often on hill pastures that are not economic for other farming methods, and only in severe winter weather do they need extra feeding stuff, and as a rule only at lambing time do they need shelter.

Pork

All the pork eaten in Britain is home bred. The pig has been a popular animal for meat for hundreds of years probably because it was easy to feed on beech mast and acorns and on domestic food waste. Nowadays, like all meat animals,

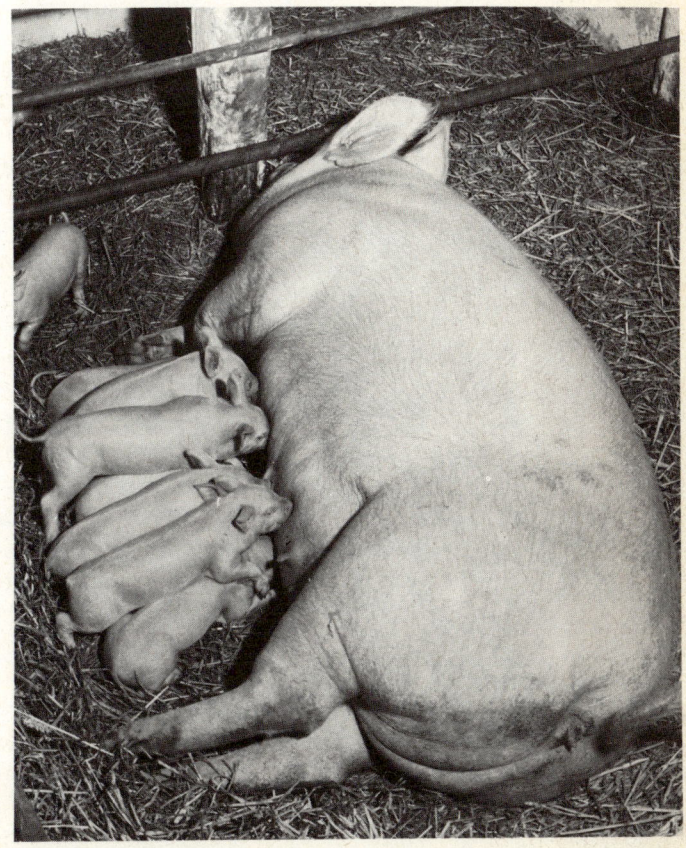

Large white pig

pigs are carefully bred to produce the right shape and most carefully fed to bring them to the right weight of 100 to 130 lb (45·5 to 59 kg) at about four months old. The food for pigs must not contain too much roughage and on first, gradual weaning they are given concentrated pig pellets and then a diet of cereal and skimmed milk with supplements of protein and minerals. There is no rooting in the woods or wallowing in a shabby sty for modern pigs—they are housed in airy, damp-proof houses kept at a temperature of 15°–20°C (60°–70°F) and in these hygienic quarters they keep very clean, as is their natural inclination.

The British breeds used to produce very large pigs but nowadays cross breeding has evolved smaller pigs without too much fat. One British breed, the Large White, is crossed with another, the Wessex Saddleback; Wessex and Essex Saddlebacks are crossed to give the new British Saddleback. Several breeds from abroad have been introduced, one from U.S.A.—the Hampshire has proved its worth; some others are more recent arrivals and they have not yet proved their value.

Not many years ago it was considered unwise to eat pork when there is no R in the month. This was because the pork readily became tainted in warm weather; nowadays the hygiene of pig-keeping and of butchers' cold stores is so good that pork is safe to eat all the year round.

Bacon

Pigs that are to be used for bacon are reared rather differently from 'porkers' as bacon-curing factories are most exact in their requirements. The bacon pig must have a long back to give plenty of back bacon, well developed hind legs and lightly built shoulders and it must not be too fat. Perhaps this exact demand is one of the reasons why Britain does not produce all the bacon we eat, the other is probably the very great competition from Danish bacon.

As for porkers the breed of pig is important for good bacon pigs. Three popular breeds now are the Landrace, which has been imported from Sweden and which has the right long-backed, light-shouldered shape; the native Wessex Saddleback, or a cross between Landrace and Large White. Danish bacon is almost entirely from Landrace pigs.

The bacon pig is fed, housed and tended as carefully as the porker but it lives rather longer—up to 6 to 8 months old

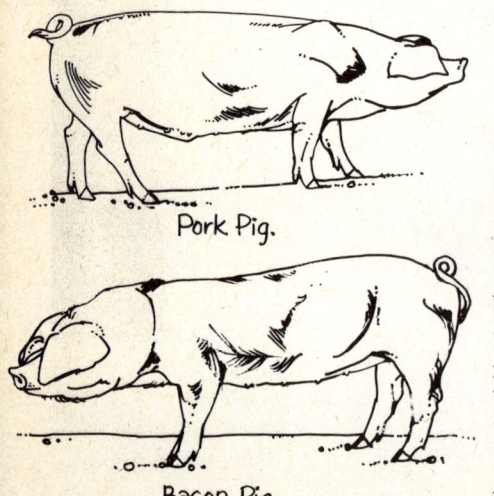

Pork Pig.

Bacon Pig.

or until it reaches 200 lb (90 kg) or for high quality lean bacon 150 to 180 lb (68 to 81·5 kg). It must not be too fat and it must not have drunk too much water or the flesh will be soft.

Bacon is 'cured' or salted and some of it is also smoked. This was originally done on the farm but is now an exact factory process. After slaughter the carcase is bled, scalded and scraped to remove bristles and then weighed and inspected. The head, trotters, internal organs and internal fat are removed —not, of course, to be wasted. The undercut of the loin is filleted out and the shoulderblade bone removed. The carcase is cut into two sides, dry salt is packed into bone cavities and brine injected into the fleshier parts. The sides are now immersed in tanks of brine where they remain for at least four days. Next they are stacked in a maturing room, kept at a cool 5°C (40°F) for one or two weeks.

If the bacon is to be sold unsmoked or green it is now ready. For smoking the sides are hung from hooks in the smoke room to dry, then oak or deal sawdust is lit and allowed to smoulder under them for 36 to 60 hours. The temperature throughout the smoking must not rise above 38°C (100°F) or the bacon would begin to cook. Smoking alters the flavour of bacon but not the keeping quality.

Hams are cut from the carcase before curing, cut with a rounded top and are cured and smoked separately often with a special recipe. If the hind legs are left on and smoked as part of the side they are known as gammon.

POULTRY

The term poultry is used to include chickens, turkeys, ducks, geese and, more rarely, guinea fowl. Except ducks and geese these birds were brought to this country from other parts of the world; chickens from Asia, turkeys from North America and guinea fowl, originally called turkey cocks or hens, came from Turkey.

Chickens

Before the second world war poultry rearing was often a sideline on a mixed farm, managed by the farmer's wife; the birds were allowed to scratch about in the farm yard and to glean in the harvest field as well as being well fed on corn and mash. There were also specialised poultry farms but the industry was small and chicken was then a dish for a rather special occasion. During the war the right food was scarce and dear because ships could not spare space for any but food for human beings and all homegrown cereals were rationed. These difficulties made farmers realise the value of poultry. After the war poultry farming started again on a much larger scale and it has continued to grow up to the present time, so that now it is an enormous industry, producing all the chickens (and eggs) that we can eat, at prices lower than that of most meat.

In order to keep the price low and the quality of the chickens high the birds, like the larger meat animals, must be bred selectively and fed on just the right amount and kind of food. The aim is now to produce birds of uniform weight of from 3 to $3\frac{1}{2}$ lb (1·3 to 1·5 kg) in 9 to 10 weeks and this is achieved by breeding birds that form flesh quickly on light-boned frames and convert the food they eat readily into flesh. As well as breeding and feeding housing must be economical as well as hygienic and labour costs must be kept low. The houses are arranged so that one worker can look after 10,000 to 20,000 birds and as each

Below *'Broiler' chicken breeding unit*
Above right *Dressing poultry*
Below right *Packing poultry*

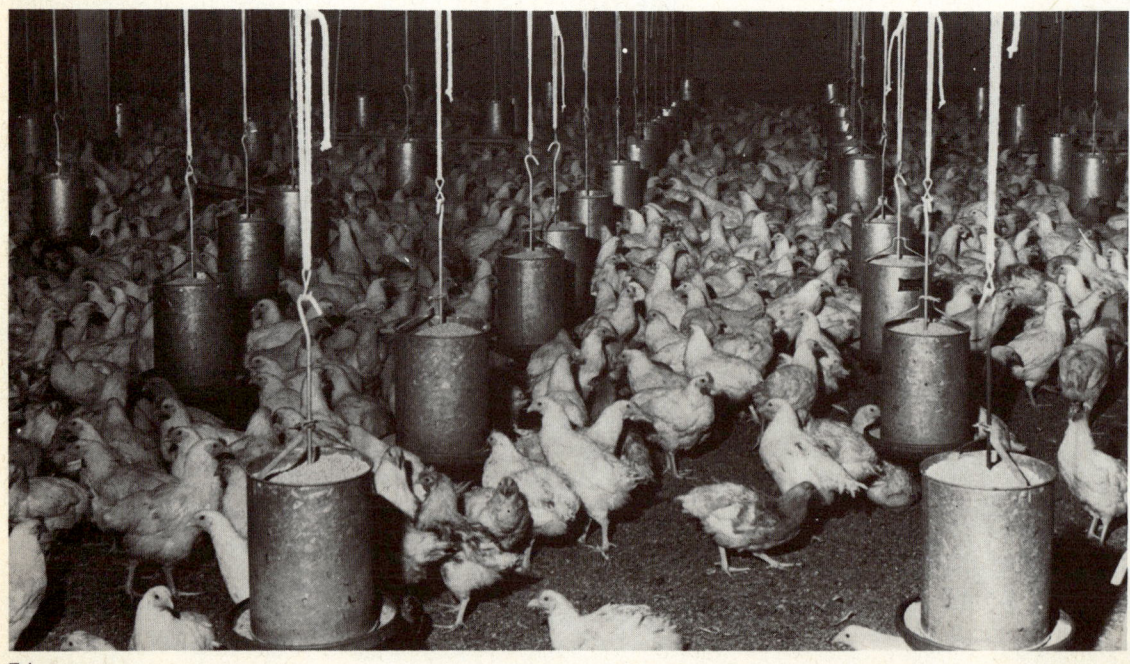

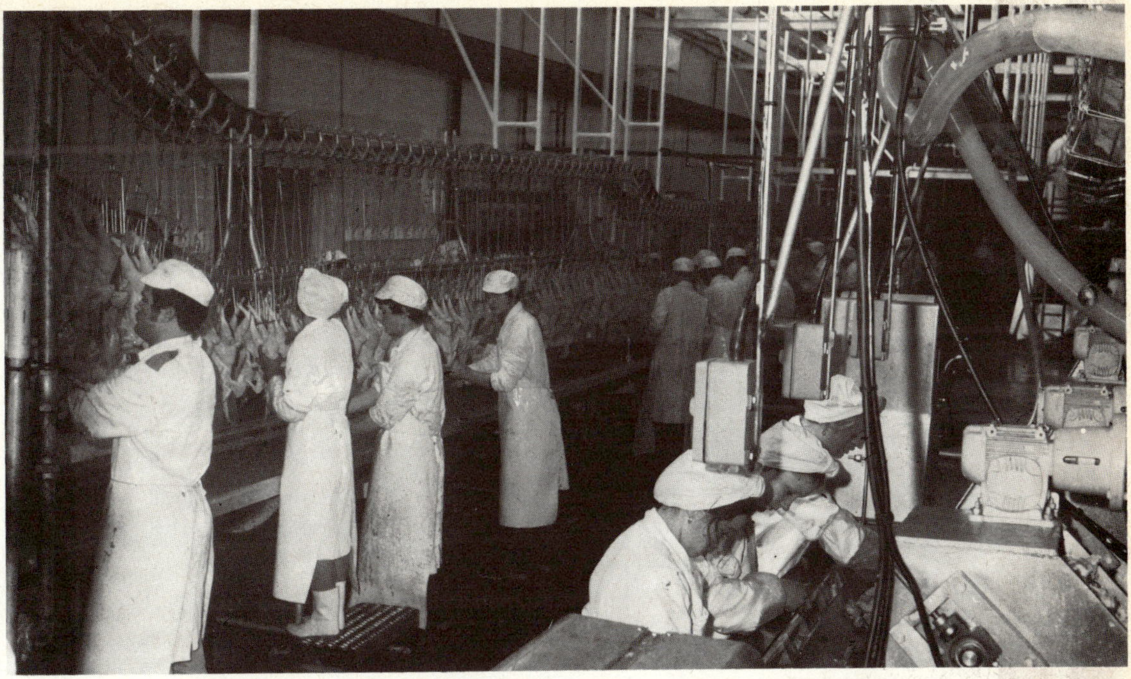

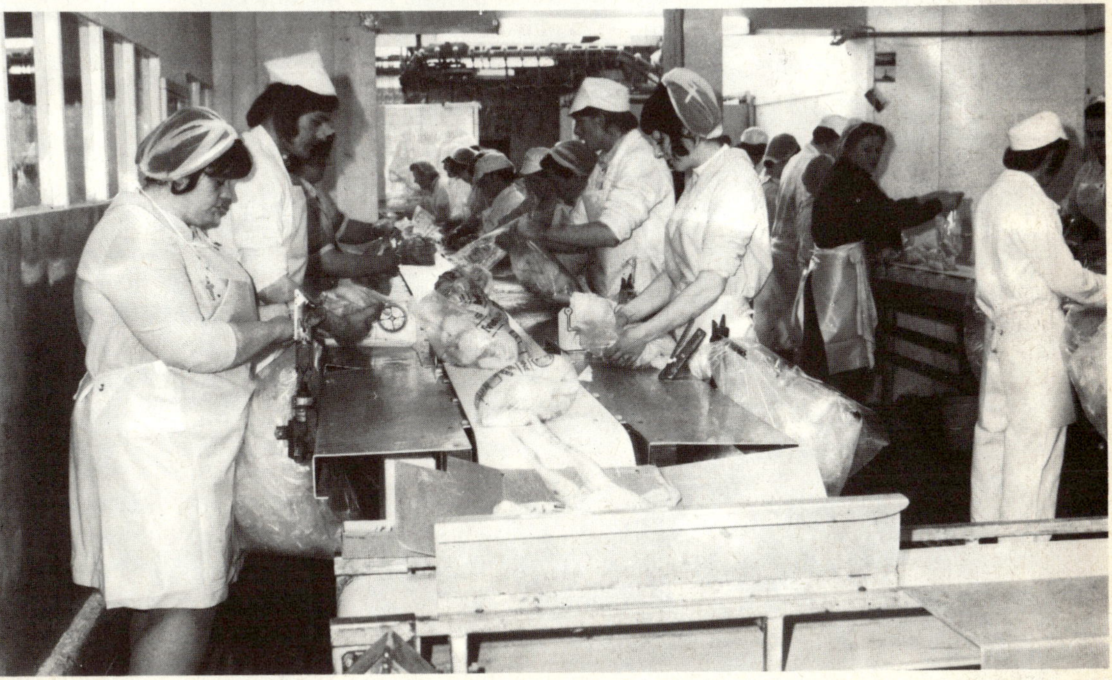

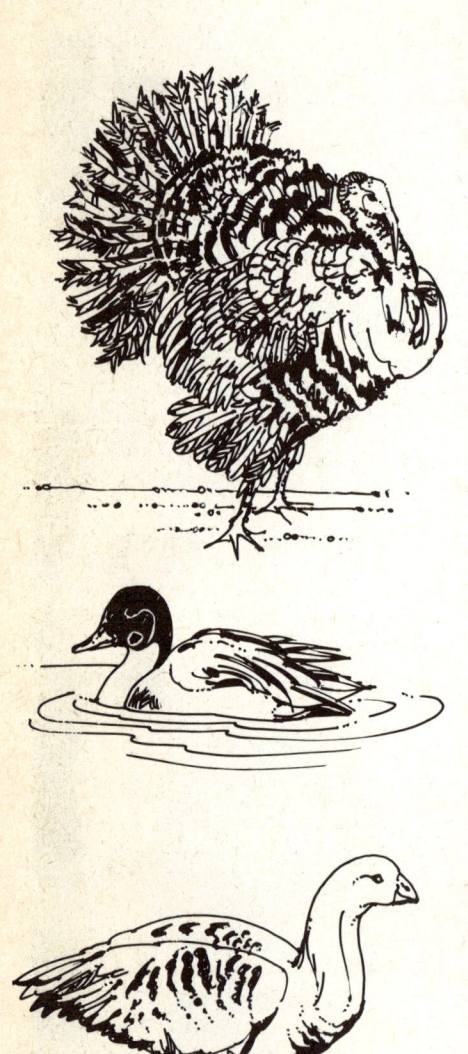

batch of birds only occupies the house for ten weeks, four batches can be raised in a year; allowing two weeks between batches for cleaning and disinfecting the house.

These young birds are known as young roasters or 'broilers' (broiling is American for grilling) which means that they can be cooked by grilling or frying as well as roasting and they are mainly intended for deep freezing. The larger birds which you see in the shops, usually not frozen, are probably the cockerels from an egg-laying flock, reared to a heavier weight often on free range. The broilers are killed, plucked by machines, cleaned, chilled, packed in film and then quick frozen, at a packing station which may or may not belong to the producer.

Turkeys

The turkey industry is not as large as that for broiler chickens but it has grown enormously in the last twenty years and rather on the same lines as chicken farming. Breeding has developed smaller, plumper birds than the traditional Christmas dinner monster, although, of course, there is still a demand for large birds at Christmas. A turkey can now weigh as little as 6 pounds but 8 to 10 lb (2·7, 3·6 and 4·5 kg) is more usual. A turkey farm if anything needs more careful management than a broiler unit because the birds are more delicate when young and of course more costly.

Ducks

Ducks are not reared in such large numbers as chickens but the industry is growing fast. They are as yet more expensive than chickens and their size is deceptive as there is not a great depth of flesh on their rather large bone structure. They are delicious to eat. They are usually sold at three to four months old when they are really still ducklings. Many of them are deep frozen like broilers.

Geese

Fewer geese are reared and sold even than ducks. They are much larger birds but have the same disadvantage of comparatively little flesh on large frames. From three to four months old they are called 'green geese' and at six to seven months old they weigh from 7 to 10 lb (3·1 to 4·5 kg). Production of geese is not growing as fast as that of turkeys.

Eggs

Although eggs as a food are quite distinct from chickens, egg production is a part of the poultry industry but nowadays usually a separate part as most large poultry units market either young roasters or eggs but not both. Some egg units, mainly small ones, rear cockerels for the table as a sideline.

The same scientific breeding as in the table poultry industry is used to develop a race of hens that will lay the maximum number of eggs for the minimum of food. The housing of the laying birds, usually in battery cages, is so arranged that feeding, watering, cleaning and egg collection can be done with the minimum of labour. This is because we all want eggs at a reasonable price and therefore management cost must be kept low if the unit owner is to make a

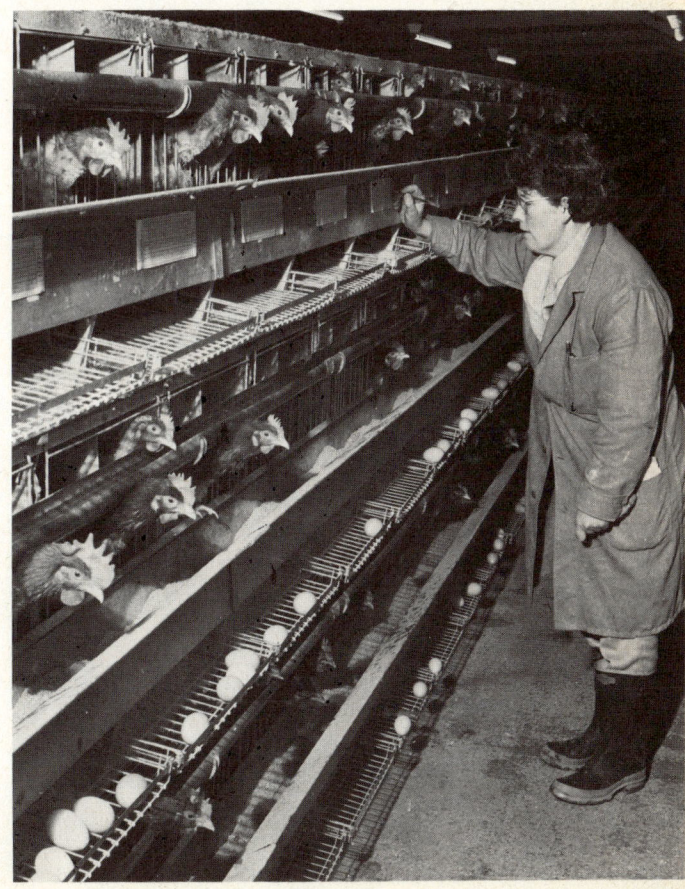

Battery cages

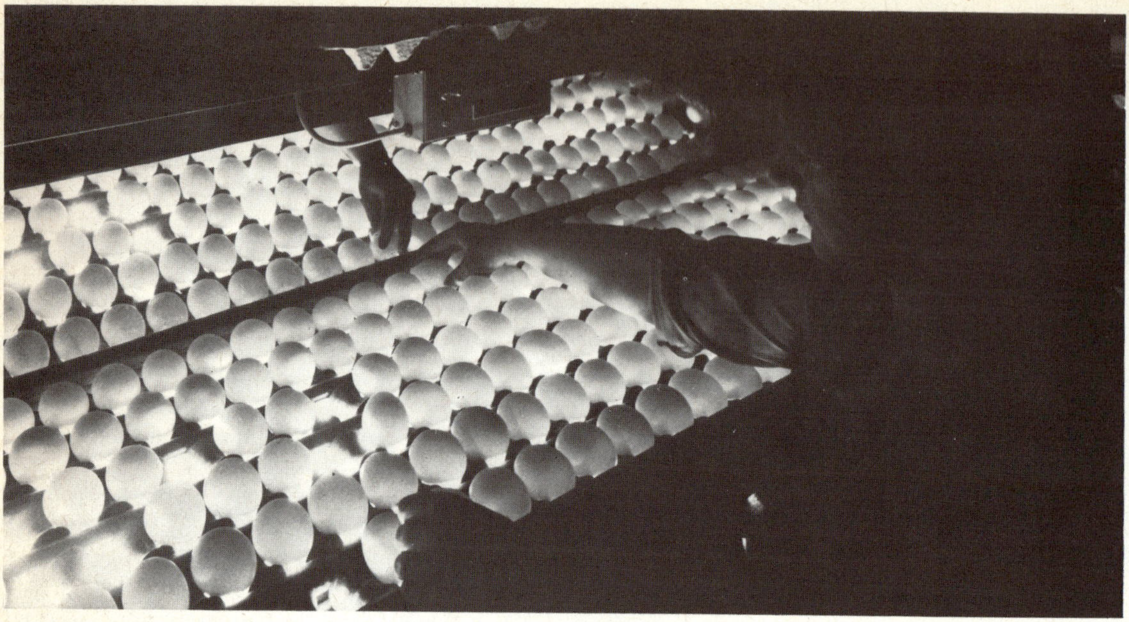

Candling

Grading and packing

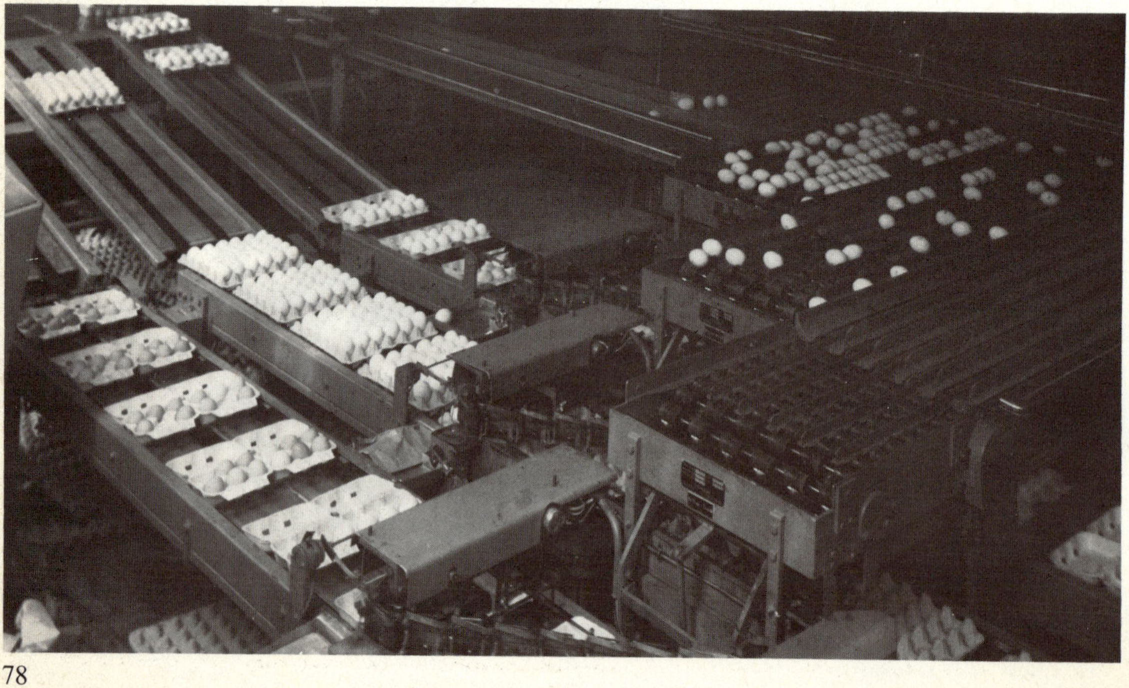

Egg Quality

The following quality classes are requirements laid down by EEC regulations enforceable as from 1st February 1973:

Class A (First Quality)

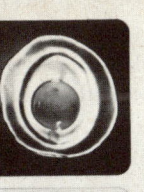
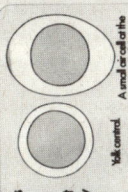

Excellent internal quality and has three distinct parts: the yolk (visible under candling as a clear translucent shadow only), a clear translucent white of a gelatinous consistency and an outer layer of thin white.

Yolk central

A small air cell at the broad end of the egg

Class B (Second Quality)

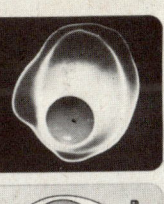
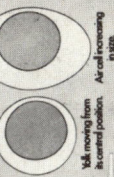

Fair internal quality. The yolk flattening, the two layers of white mingling.

Yolk moving from its central position

Air cell increasing in size

Class C (Third Quality)

They are suitable for the manufacture of foodstuffs for human consumption. Includes all eggs which do not satisfy the requirements of the first two classes.

Wallchart No. 2.

Published by the British Egg Information Service, Haymarket House, Oxendon Street, London SW1Y 4EW

THE EP GROUP OF COMPANIES

Egg weight grades

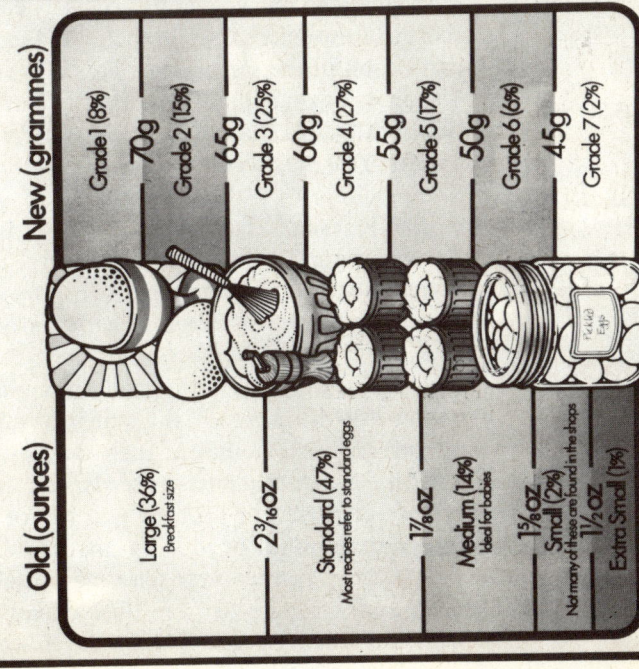

Old (ounces)	New (grammes)
Large (36%) Breakfast size	Grade 1 (8%) — 70g
	Grade 2 (15%) — 65g
2³/₁₆oz	Grade 3 (25%) — 60g
Standard (47%) Most recipes refer to standard eggs	Grade 4 (27%) — 55g
1⅞oz	Grade 5 (17%) — 50g
Medium (14%) Ideal for babies	Grade 6 (6%) — 45g
1⅝oz Small (2%)	Grade 7 (2%)
1½oz Extra Small (1%) Not many of these are found in the shops	

This chart is a comparison of the existing weight grades for the United Kingdom and those in use in the European Economic Community.

There are seven grades for Class A and B eggs. (Class relates to quality standards. Class C eggs need not be weight graded.

The figure shown in brackets is the grade's estimated % share of total production.

Published by the British Egg Information Service, Haymarket House, Oxendon Street, London SW1Y 4EW

Wallchart No. 5.

THE EP GROUP OF COMPANIES

profit. Hens in nature, like all birds, lay their eggs in the spring so, in order to ensure a steady supply of eggs all the year round, the lighting and warming of the houses has to simulate perpetual spring so that egg laying does not decrease with seasonal changes of length of daylight and of temperature. Britain can now produce all the eggs needed for domestic consumption all the year round; some are imported for bakery and manufacturing use.

At a packing station the eggs are cleaned (not washed as this makes the shell liable to absorb infection), tested for freshness and strength of shell and for the absence of any faults such as blood spots which are harmless but look unattractive. They are graded into the sizes we know in the shops and sometimes for brown or white shells (some people will pay more for brown shelled eggs although the food value is the same as the white ones) and are then packed in cases for dispatch to the retailer. Some eggs are sold at the farm or a farm shop.

MILK

As you know, a cow, before she can give milk, must first have a calf, so dairy farming is closely connected with stock rearing although the two branches of farming are not always carried on in the same farm. This is because breeding over hundreds of years has evolved some cattle that are good for beef and others that give a high milk yield with a few dual breeds. You may recognise some of the famous dairy breeds. They include:
British Friesian, black and white and also good for beef,
Ayrshires, dark brown and white,
Dairy Shorthorns, many mixtures of brown, white and roan,
Jersey, small, fawn coloured with sooty rings round their eyes,
Guernseys, light tan with some white patches.

Some of these breeds, the Friesians and Shorthorns, and others not listed above, such as Red Polls and South Devons, are dual purpose breeds, in other words the male calves are reared or sold for rearing for beef, and the cow calves are kept for producing calves and milk.

The dairy farmer first selects a suitable breed of dairy cows and arranges to have their calves fathered by a bull with a record of daughters who have given high milk

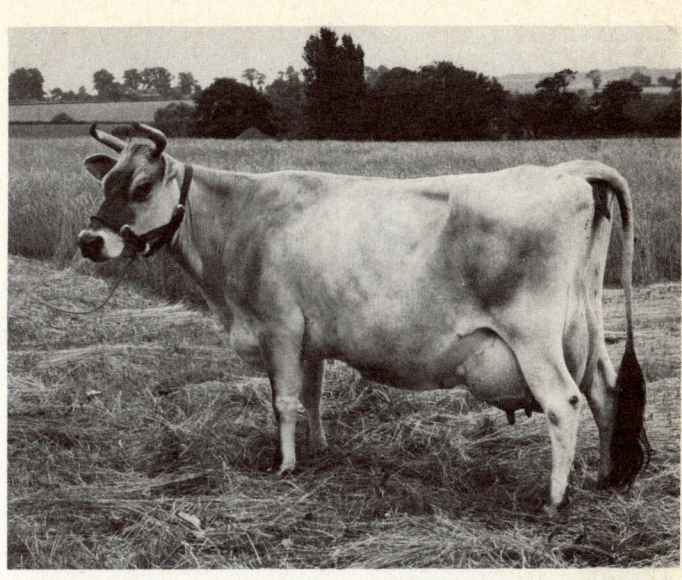

Jersey cow

yields, nowadays this is often done by artificial insemination. Then he must feed the herd correctly on good pasturage or silage with supplements of other foods especially before calving and during lactation. The food for a dairy cow may be rationed by a computer.

When the calf is born the mother cow feeds it for only a few days and then it is hand-reared on plenty of milk, with other foods gradually added. A cow bred for milking gives far more milk than her calf needs, so a little is saved for the calf and the rest is sold.

Milking is nowadays almost always done by machinery, often in a milk parlour or even a rotary unit, in both of which the cows stand in stalls on a raised platform so the milker can easily fix the suction cups of the milking machine to the cows' teats. Everything used during milking must be spotlessly clean; the milker's clothing, the floor and furniture and of course every part of the machinery. The cow's udder is first washed with a spray of warm water. The machine draws the milk either into a closed bucket, a glass container or into a churn, in either case it is strained and the milk from each cow is weighed for the record. The milk is next run over a cooler and then emptied into churns or into a large tank. If the milk is already in a churn, the churn is cooled. It is then ready for transport to the nearest bottling centre or transferred to tankers for transport by

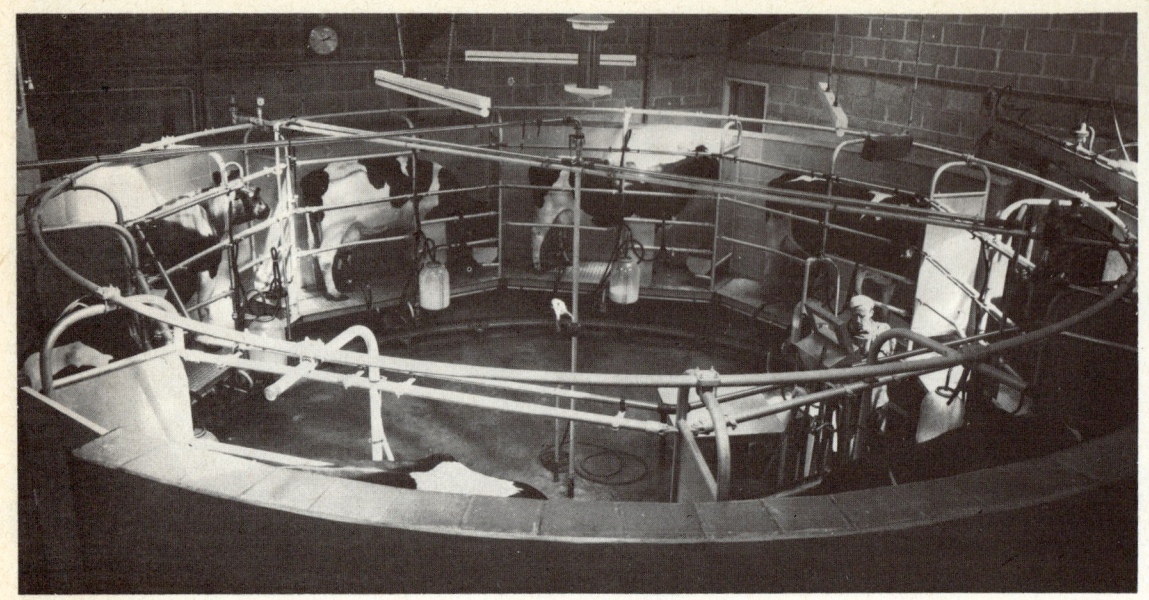

Modern milking carousel (rotary unit)

road or rail to bottling centres in large towns. Within one day after milking the milk must be tested for freshness by an expert 'sniffer', pasteurised, cooled, bottled and sent to the distributing dairy. Meanwhile samples of milk are tested in a laboratory of the bottling plant for fat content, solids-not-fat content and for the number of bacteria. Some of the tests are made before and some after pasteurising.

All dairy herds in Britain are now free of tuberculosis, and to keep this state of affairs they are regularly given a tuberculin test. Any cows that do not pass the test are withdrawn from the herd. Other treatments given to some milk are homogenisation, by which the milk is put under pressure to divide up the fat into minute globules; sterilisation by heat so that the milk, if unopened, will keep for one or two weeks, and ultra heat treatment (U.H.T.) to well above boiling point so that the milk, if kept sealed, will be in good condition one or two months later, without refrigeration. The latest scientific aim is to have all dairy herds certified as free of brucellosis—a disease which can affect human beings as well as cows.

Cream

Milk is separated at a creamery into cream and skimmed milk. The milk is warmed to 32°C (90°F) and then spun in a centrifugal separator at 6,000 revolutions a minute. The cream is flung to the top and drawn off at a regulated percentage of butter fat—18 per cent for single cream, 48 per cent for double cream or 35 to 40 per cent for butter-making. The cream is next cooled then pasteurised at 79·5°C (175°F) for fresh cream or at a lower 60°C (140°F) for butter-making.

The skimmed milk is drawn off from the separator by a different pipe from that used for the cream and is pasteurised. It is then sent away to be used for animal feeding, for drying as powdered milk, for other low fat milk products or even for plastics manufacture.

Butter

In Britain we import 88 per cent of the butter we eat, making only 12 per cent, probably because only about 4 per cent of milk is fat, and it therefore takes a great deal of milk to make a worthwhile amount of butter. After the cream has been separated (see under cream) it is kept overnight, then *Butter making* churned for some 40 minutes till it has formed little granules.

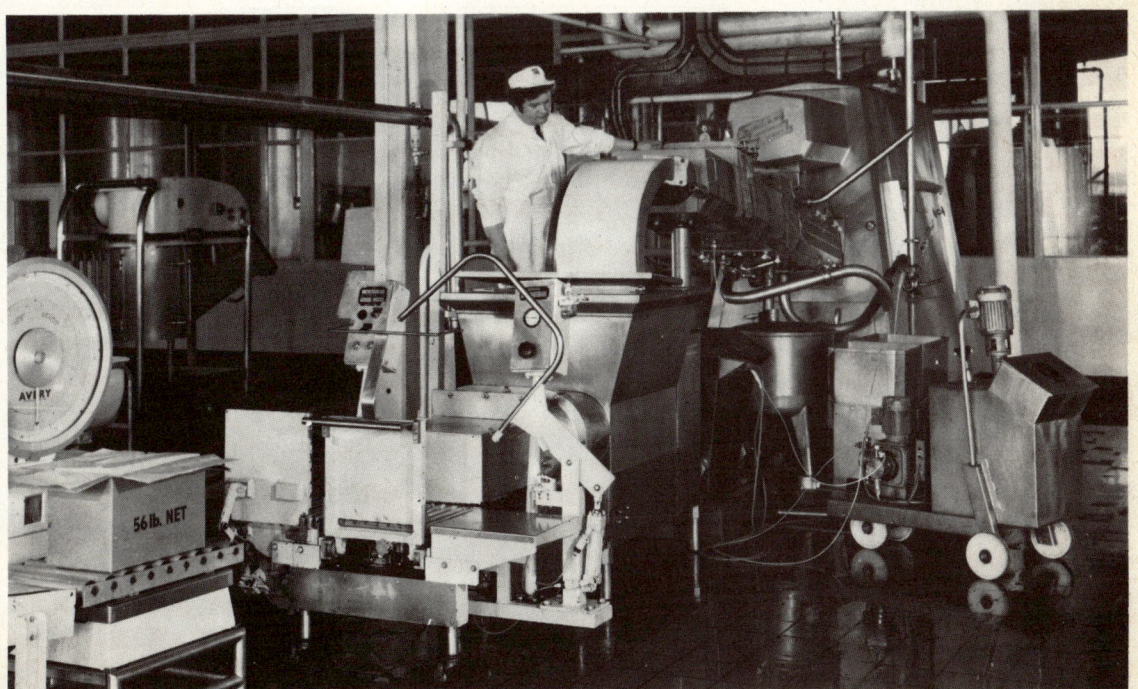

At this stage the buttermilk is drawn off and the butter is washed in the churn with chilled water. Salt is then worked in evenly at which stage the butter is a smooth mass and ready for packing in large boxes or in the weighed half-pound packets in which we buy it.

The buttermilk is not wasted; it may be used for animal feeding, for making 'whey butter', for various manufacturing processes and a little of it is sold in dairies.

Other milk products are made in small quantities, for example soured cream, yoghurt, evaporated, condensed and dried milk, both skimmed and whole milk.

Cheese

We import into Britain a great deal of cheese; from Canada, New Zealand and Australia we get cheeses from recipes and methods which originated in Britain, while from Denmark, Holland, France and Switzerland we get a very wide variety of cheeses produced only in those countries, and from the United States we mostly get processed cheese:

Some of the best known British cheeses are Cheddar, Cheshire, Double Gloucester, Stilton, Wensleydale. You

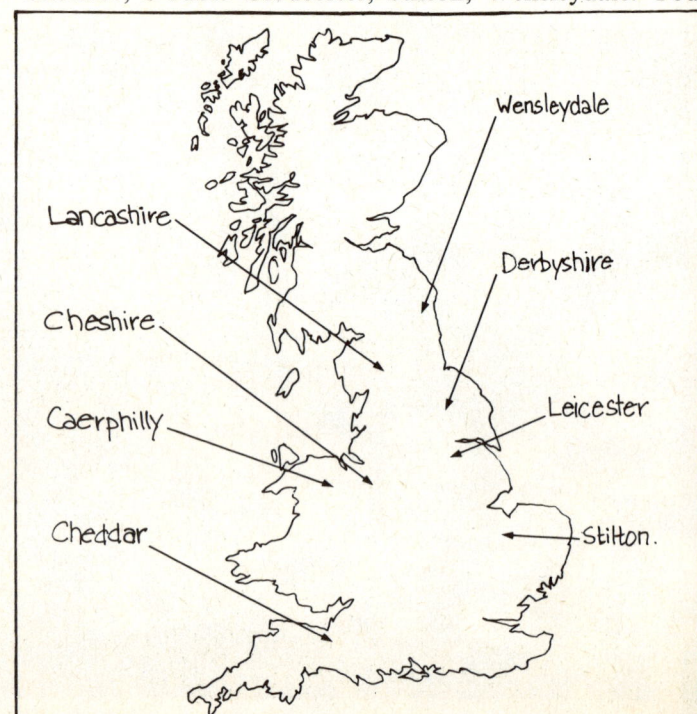

can find the names of others less well known. Originally cheese was given the name of the county or district in which it was made but nowadays a 'starter' or culture of the right cheese-forming bacteria is used and this, together with the method peculiar to the district of origin, gives the characteristic flavour and texture implied in the name. For example, 'Cheddar' cheese can be made in Canada, Australia, New Zealand or Scotland. Some cheese is still made in farms in the original districts.

Roughly the general method of making cheese is to mix milk from two days' milking, store it for some twelve hours then to add 'starter', which sours the milk because bacteria change the milk sugar to acid. Next rennet is added to solidify the milk. The curd, when it is formed, is cut into squares and some of the whey can be drained off. Next the curd is warmed to 36°C (98°F) and stirred for up to 1½ hours; this releases the rest of the whey (90 per cent of the milk) which is drawn off to be used to make 'whey butter', to be used for animal feeding or for drying for manufacturing. The curd is cut into blocks, piled up and turned continually for about two hours, it may then be ground finely before

Below *Cheese making—rennetting*
Below right *Draining the curd*

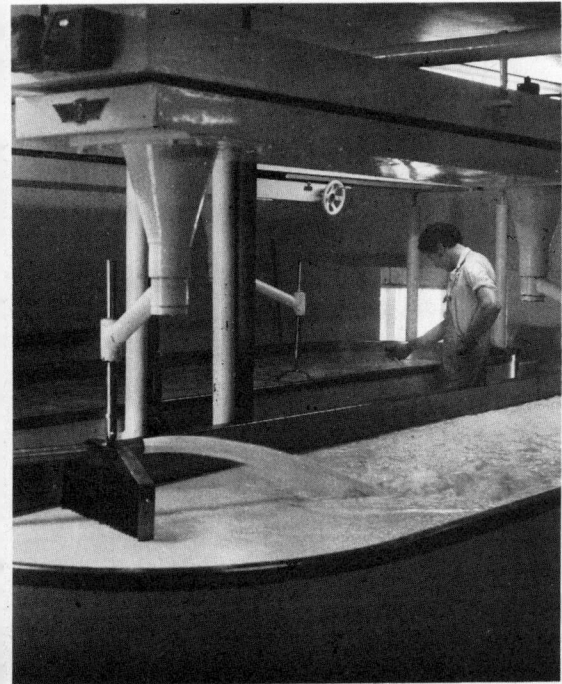
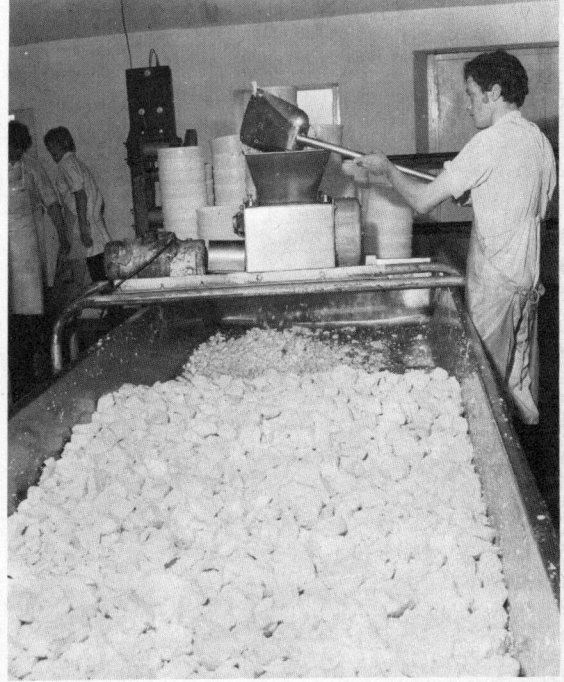

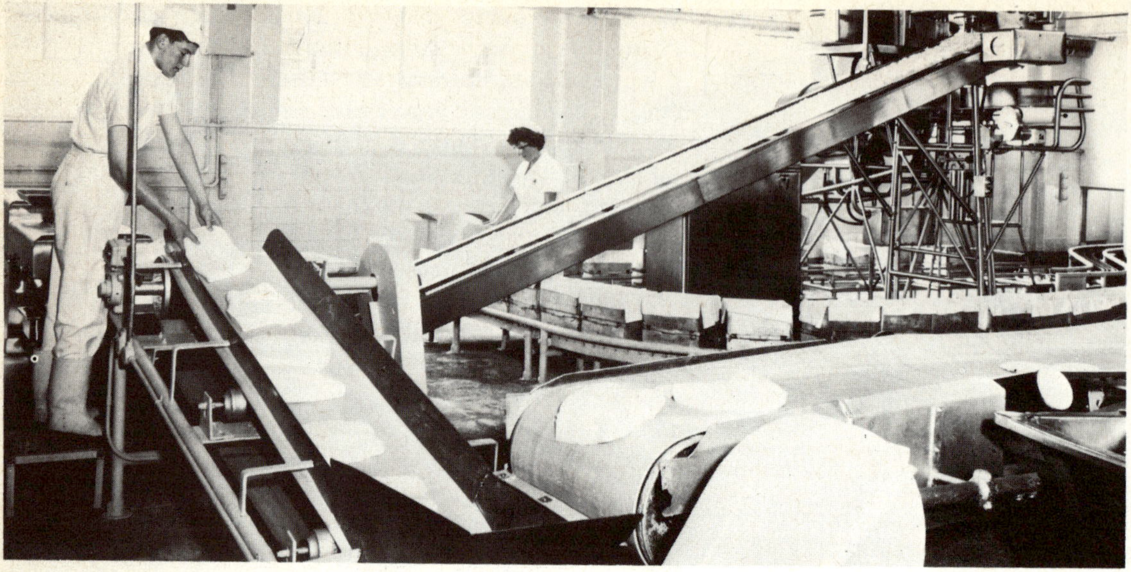

Cut curd on the way to the dicing mill

Binding and moulding cheese

Testing maturity of cheese

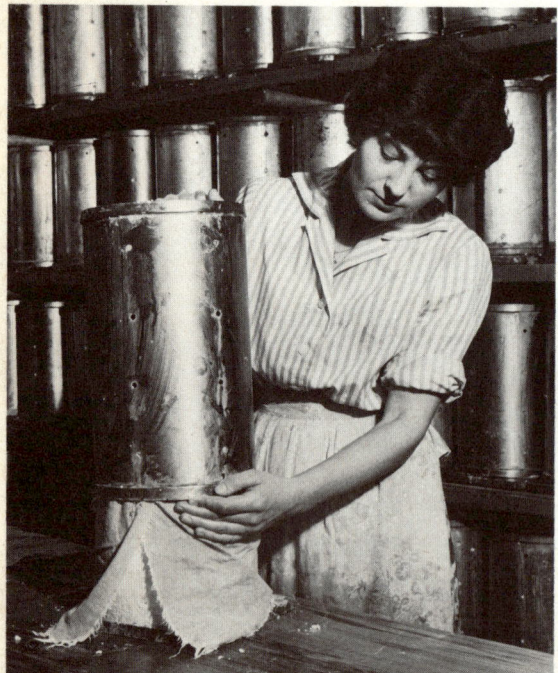

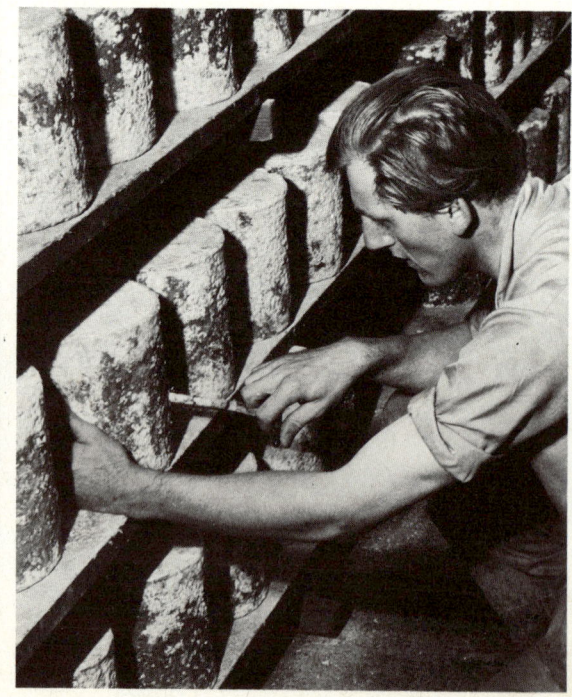

moulding and pressing. The cheeses must next ripen for a varying length of time according to their kind, but always at a temperature of about 10°C (50°F) and in a well ventilated, spotlessly clean room where humidity is carefully controlled and where they are turned over every day. When an expert cheese taster decides they are ripe and ready they are sold. The time needed for ripening varies from a few weeks to several months according to the type of cheese.

The above method is the outline for the making of Cheddar cheese; there are many variations of this method for different types of cheese.

Other milk products

As well as the various designations of liquid milk, cream, butter and cheese, milk is dried, whole (mainly for baby foods) or skimmed (for general use) because this keeps better than whole dried milk in which the fat tastes rancid after prolonged storage. Condensed milk is heat-treated and has sugar added to preserve it and milk is also evaporated to remove some of the water content and both these varieties are sealed in cans.

FISH

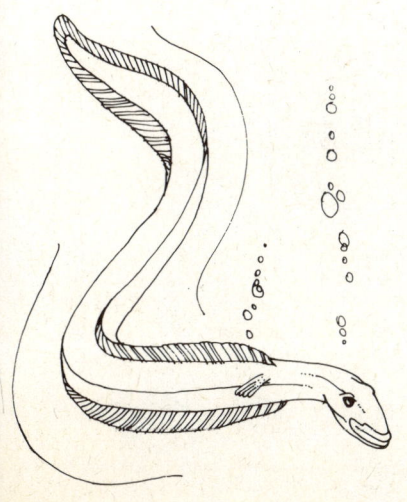

Fish differ from meat animals in that they are not domesticated—not fed and tended by man. They remain 'wild'. There are fish farms but they are mainly concerned with stocking rivers with trout or oyster beds with oysters or with research into the feeding and development of young fish and the effect on them of changing conditions in their watery environment.

Fish must be caught either in the sea or in rivers. Many freshwater fish are caught only for sport and, with the exception of eels, trout and salmon, few of them are sold in retail shops. In any case, eels, sea-trout and salmon spend part of their life at sea and only part in rivers.

Sea-fish are caught by different methods according to their way of life. If they live mainly on the sea bed, that is if they are *demersal*, they are caught in *trawl nets* dragged along the sea bed by boats called trawlers; if they swim nearer the surface, that is if they are *pelagic*, they are caught in *drift nets* which hang vertically in the water attached to two boats or a boat and a buoy and in which

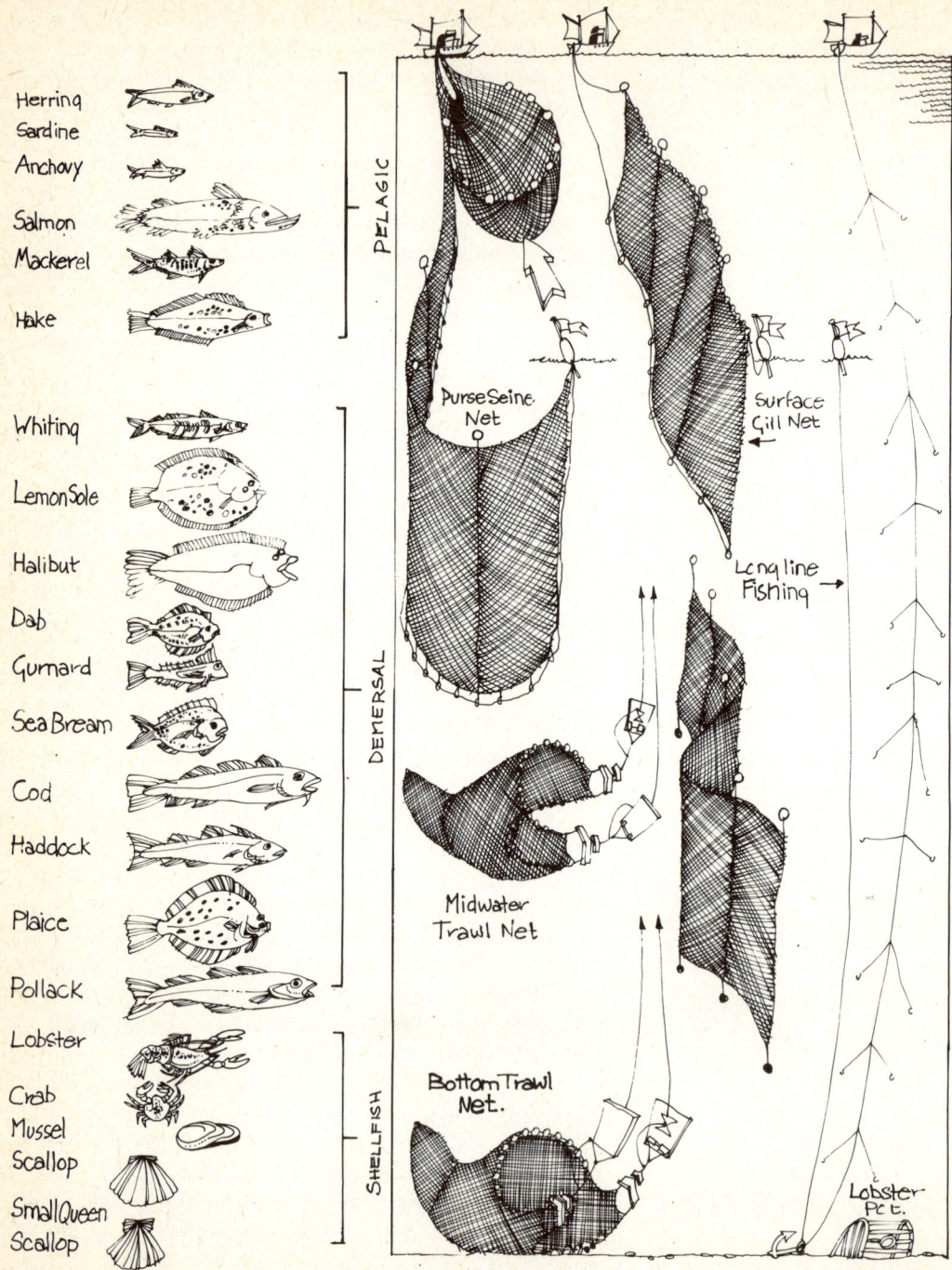

Herring
Sardine
Anchovy
Salmon
Mackerel
Hake

PELAGIC

Whiting
Lemon Sole
Halibut
Dab
Gurnard
Sea Bream
Cod
Haddock
Plaice
Pollack

DEMERSAL

Lobster
Crab
Mussel
Scallop
Small Queen Scallop

SHELLFISH

Purse Seine Net

Surface Gill Net

Long line Fishing →

Midwater Trawl Net

Bottom Trawl Net.

Lobster Pot.

the fish enmesh themselves. A *purse-seine* net is also used for catching pelagic fish; the boat circles, drawing a net round the shoal of fish and the net is then drawn tight at the bottom and hauled aboard. For salmon caught in the sea a *gill-net* is used; this has a coarse mesh in which the fish get entangled and the net is weighted at the bottom and suspended from floats between the boat and a buoy and may extend for a quarter-mile. *Line fishing* is also used for large pelagic fish such as halibut; this consists of a line hung below the surface of the sea from floats and baited at intervals on hooks.

River fish are caught by rod and line used with considerable skill or patience. Eels are usually caught in conical wicker traps, and salmon, in some rivers, are trapped or netted, often illegally.

Shellfish are caught by methods varying according to their ability to move. Crustaceans, that is crabs and lobsters, are caught in wicker traps called pots, dropped to the sea bed and marked with floats, or if they are small they may be trawled off the sea bed or scooped up by nets pushed along in shallow water by wading men. Most molluscs, because they cannot move fast, can be scooped up by various means from the sea bed or from rocks.

Inshore fishing is carried out within a mile or so of the shore and is the strict preserve of the country owning the shore. Fishing rights often cause bitter dispute between countries who rely on deep sea fishing. Some countries claim territorial waters extending for six, twelve or even fifty miles round their coasts.

Deep-sea fishing is carried on from Britain by ships much larger than the trawlers or herring drifters that fish the North Sea, and these larger ships can stay at sea for two months at a time. They have refrigerated holds so that their catch is kept in good condition although they fish far away in the North Atlantic and almost up to the Arctic Circle.

When the boats come into their home port the fish is quickly unloaded on the fish quay and auctioned to fish traders or wholesalers who send it as rapidly as possible to their customers in large towns, to other fish markets, or to other wholesale merchants.

The fishing industry is a precarious and a highly complicated one. The quantity of fish brought in depends on many vagaries of weather and migrations of fish, and the quality

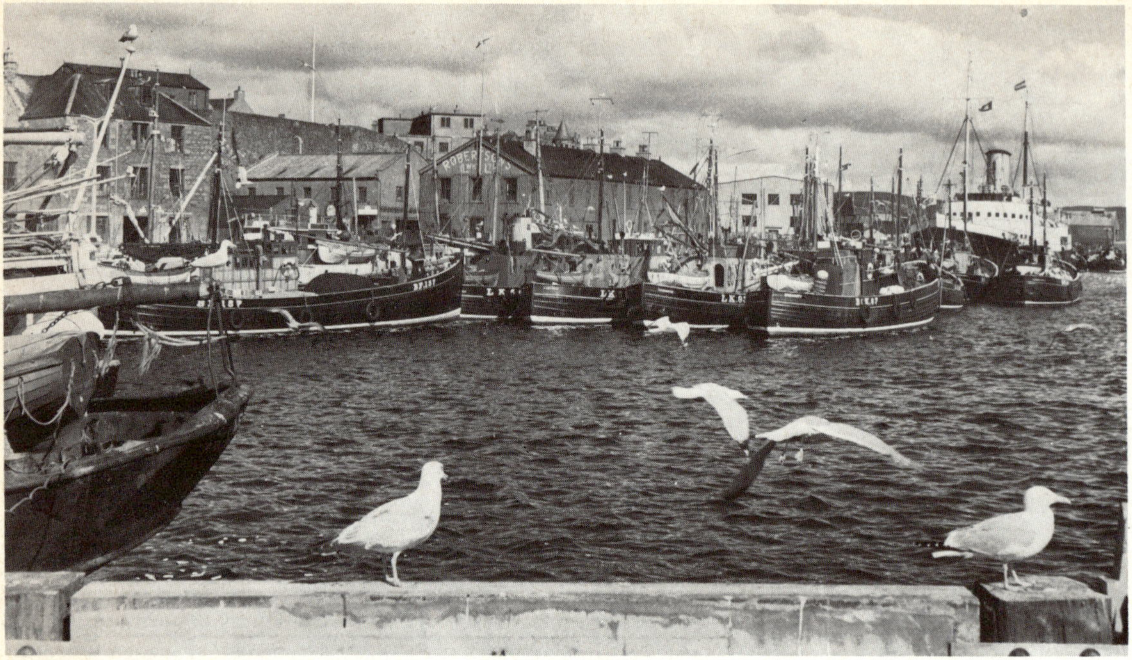

Lerwick—a busy fishing port

Angler by a river.

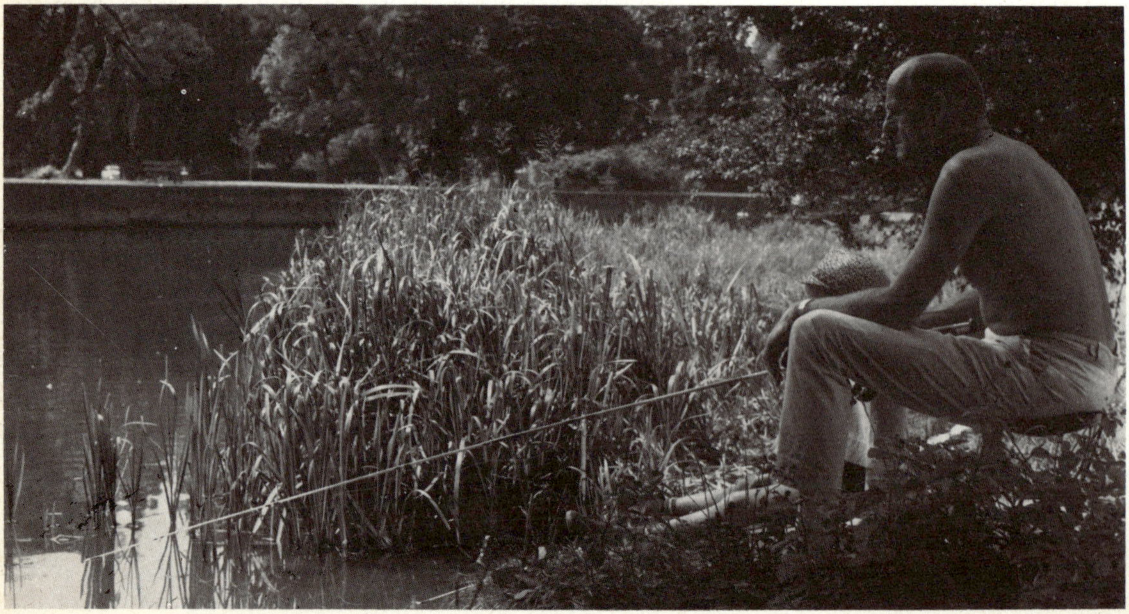

cannot be controlled as can that of farm produce. The ships and their crews have to face many hazards of storms and icy conditions at sea. As well as these difficulties fish is so highly perishable that the catch must be distributed very rapidly once it is landed.

Nowadays a large amount of the more plentiful or more popular fish is quick-frozen at factories near the fish ports so that it can be bought from any shop with a deep freeze, but for more adventurous shopping many different kinds of unusual fish appear from time to time on the fishmonger's slab. Another way of preserving fish and adding to its flavour is smoking; this is also done at or near the fishing port, as is canning. Much canned fish is imported.

VEGETABLES

Of the vegetables grown in this country more than half are grown as farm crops. These farm crops include potatoes and the brassica family, that is cabbages, brussels sprouts and cauliflowers. The growing of vegetables is carried on out of doors for the most part but the more delicate kinds are

Below *Field of cabbages*
Below right *Cucumbers in the hot house*

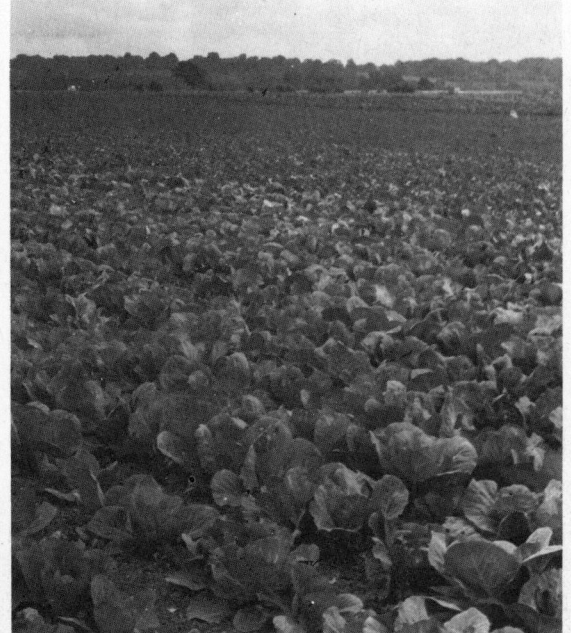
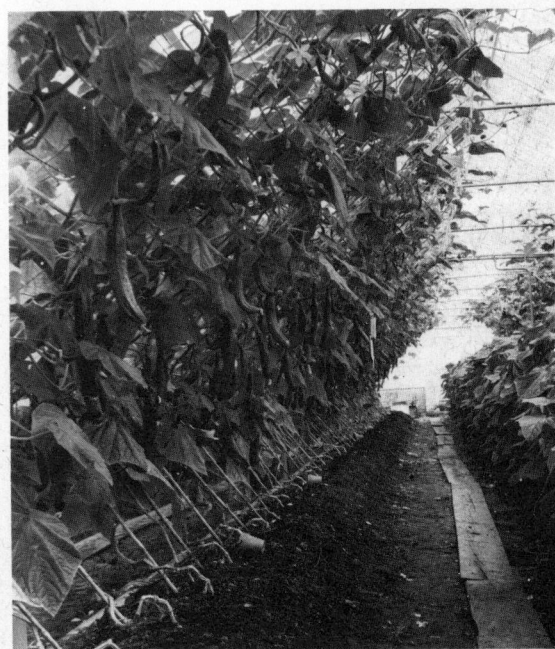

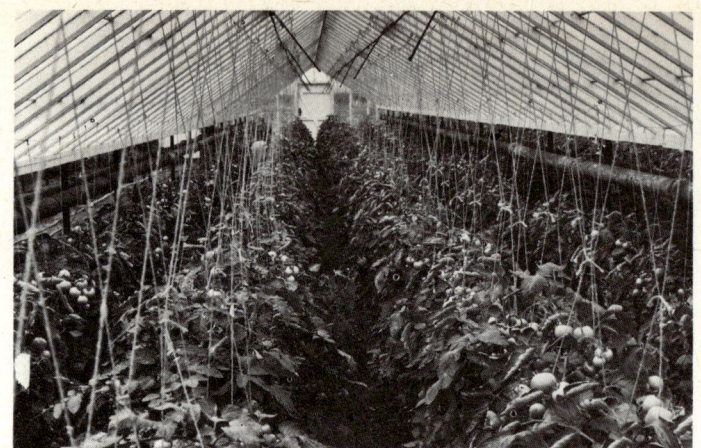

Tomatoes in a greenhouse

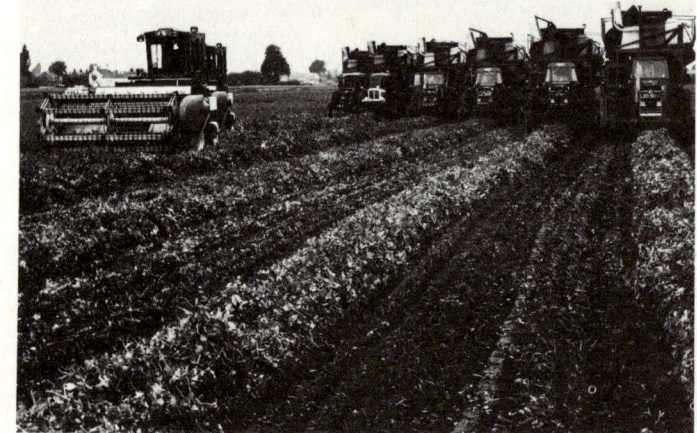

Pea harvest

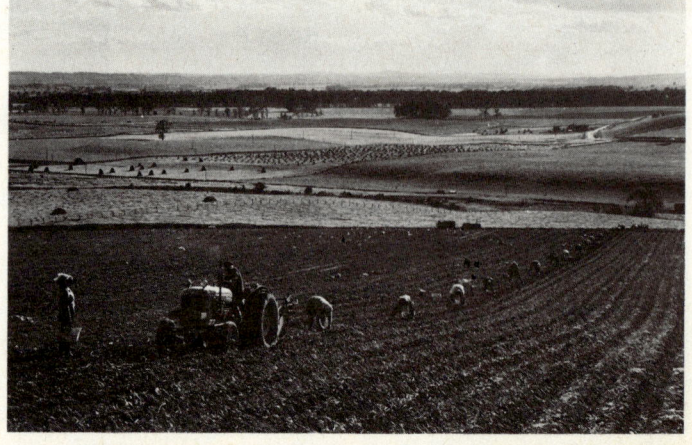

Potato harvest

grown under glass, sometimes to force them to grow out of their normal season or because they need the uniform warm temperature that our climate does not achieve.

All vegetable growing is expensive because the fertile, well drained land on which vegetables grow best is expensive, and because they need skilled care in fertilising, weeding and often staking and tying; in fact many jobs that can only be done by hand. Where machinery can be used for tilling and harvesting it is also costly.

The growing of vegetables out of doors seems to have developed as an industry for two reasons which sometimes coincide: the nearness to large towns with many customers to be fed, and the suitably fertile land. Where the land is fertile but remote from large towns efficient methods of

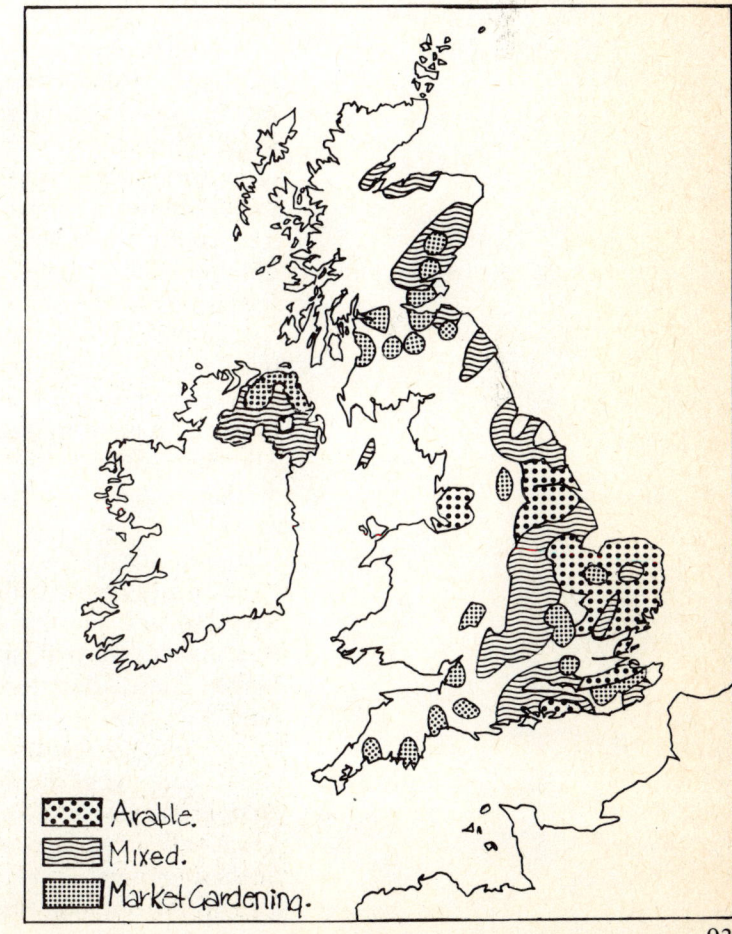

Arable.

Mixed.

Market Gardening.

transport have had to be developed. One good area for horticulture, that is vegetable and flower growing, lies conveniently all round London and another to the west of Birmingham. Two of the districts where soil and climate are right but from which large towns are distant are Cornwall and the fenlands of East Anglia.

Districts where there are many glasshouses growing vegetable and salad crops lie in the Lea Valley, probably because of its nearness to London; round Worthing because of the sunlight and the mild climate; on the Channel Islands, also for climatic reasons; in West Lancashire where the nearness to large towns is important; and in East Yorkshire because, lying as it does near to Holland many Dutch growers settled there and brought with them their traditional skills.

Although there are many small market gardens, as in farming, the units tend to grow to a very large size. One modern development has taken place because of the huge frozen food industry so that nowadays many horticulturists grow their peas, beans, spinach, broccoli, or other crops exclusively for a firm which will quick freeze and pack them. The freezer firm will advise the grower on the kind of vegetable and the volume of the crop and will supervise the fertilising and the harvesting at exactly the right time.

Like other food producing industries vegetable growing is constantly improving its techniques and its output, thanks to research into weed and pest control. Constant effort has to be and is made to restrict the use of chemicals harmful to wild life. Scientific advances have also been made in the mechanisation of such jobs as tilling and harvesting various crops.

In addition to our home production, Britain imports a large quantity of vegetables and salads from Europe, chiefly from Holland and France with some from Italy and Spain and, further abroad, from North Africa, Israel and the United States. Potatoes, unless our crops fail, we only import as 'new' from Spain, the Canaries and the Channel Islands, with a few from Cyprus. From the more distant countries some of the imports are of vegetables that never grow in Britain, or are out of season. If they are perishable and highly prized they may be brought in by air. The result of these imports is that many vegetables are never out of season, for example tomatoes; some, even if they are not imported when out of season, can probably be bought deep frozen, as for example, peas and runner beans.

The marketing of vegetable crops is complicated and the industry is even more affected by the weather and by supply and demand than is the agricultural industry. For example, good growing conditions and a bumper crop will result in a glut on the market which will cause the price to fall, but may not lead to a much greater quantity being bought by the general public. This will mean the grower will receive less money per item sold, and he may not sell much more of his bumper crop than if his crop was normal.

FRUIT

The fruit grower has much the same problems as the horticulturist but his are even greater because the trees, on which many of his crops grow, may take as long as ten years to develop fully so that, if he finds a particular type unproductive or unsaleable, he must wait a long time before he can replace it. Added to this the fruit grower faces fierce competition from abroad. Britain imports more fruit per head of population than any other country in the world, and from all over the world. Some popular imported fruits such as oranges and lemons we cannot, of course, grow in our climate except expensively under glass.

Of the fruit that can be grown in Britain apples are perhaps the most plentiful crop and, although the season is short, by storing some of the crop in specially constructed buildings where a uniform humidity and a supply of carbon-dioxide can be maintained, growers can have apples in good condition for market some months after harvesting them. However, apples are imported from all over the world—from Australia, New Zealand, South Africa, Canada, the United States and Europe, at prices comparable with those of the homegrown varieties. The story of pears and of cherries resembles that of apples, but we are more nearly self-supporting in plums and soft fruits.

Some of the homegrown soft fruits, mainly raspberries, strawberries, gooseberries and plums, are canned or made into jam in this country. We also import large quantities of canned fruits of all kinds, particularly those varieties that we cannot grow in our climate.

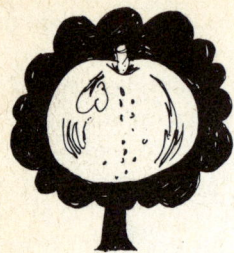

Tydeman's Early
Very like a Worcester but redder, larger, rounder and less conical in shape. It is juicy and sweet-scented.
AUGUST–SEPTEMBER.

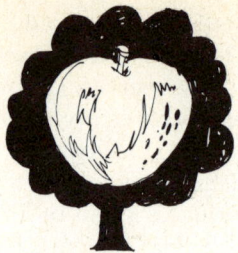

Worcester Pearmain
A rich red apple with some pale green streaks; very juicy and sweet. Worcesters should be eaten as soon as possible after purchase.
SEPTEMBER–NOVEMBER.

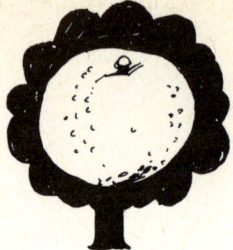

Egremont Russet
A rare, delicious apple, easy to recognise by its russet brown skin with orange blush. It is medium-sized and crisp, with a nutty flavour.
OCTOBER–DECEMBER.

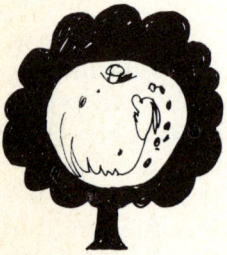

Cox's Orange Pippin
The finest-flavoured of all apples. The colour of Cox is variable usually palish green with orange to red flush; the brown russet marks around the stem are superficial and do not affect the flesh of the apple.
LATE SEPTEMBER–APRIL.

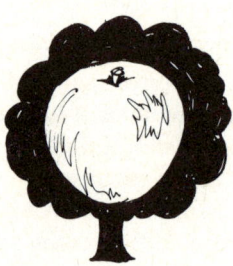

Laxton's Superb
Due to its Cox parentage, it is often mistaken for Cox's Orange Pippin. It is, however, slightly sweeter and it is the later variety.
NOVEMBER–APRIL.

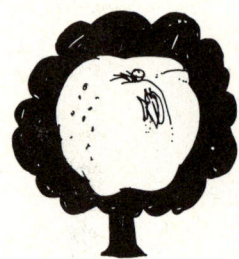

Lord Derby
Lord Derby has a distinctive shape, slightly conical with pronounced 'ribs'. A fine cooking apple which fills the gap between Grenadier and Bramleys which it resembles closely in colour.
SEPTEMBER–NOVEMBER.

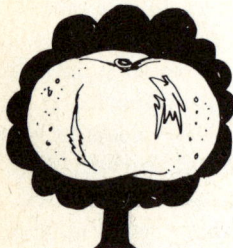

Bramley's Seedling
Bramleys are the best known of English cooking apples, are ideal for stewing and especially for baking. Have a deep green waxy skin, sometimes with a slight orange-red flush.
OCTOBER–JUNE.

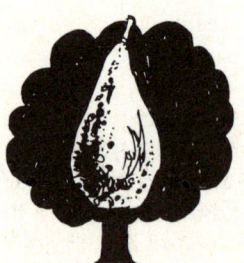

Conference
An excellent eating pear also good for cooking and bottling. It is medium-sized, with an irregular, tapering shape. Can be eaten when 'nutty' or can be ripened further at home.
OCTOBER–FEBRUARY.

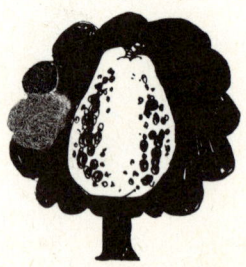

Comice
Comice has a superb flavour, being sweet and juicy under its tough skin and literally melts in the mouth.
NOVEMBER–DECEMBER.

CEREALS

The word 'cereal' is taken from the name of Ceres, the Roman goddess of the earth and of harvest, but thousands of years before the Romans worshipped her the crops to which she gave her special protection were of great importance to prehistoric men. It was not until they began to

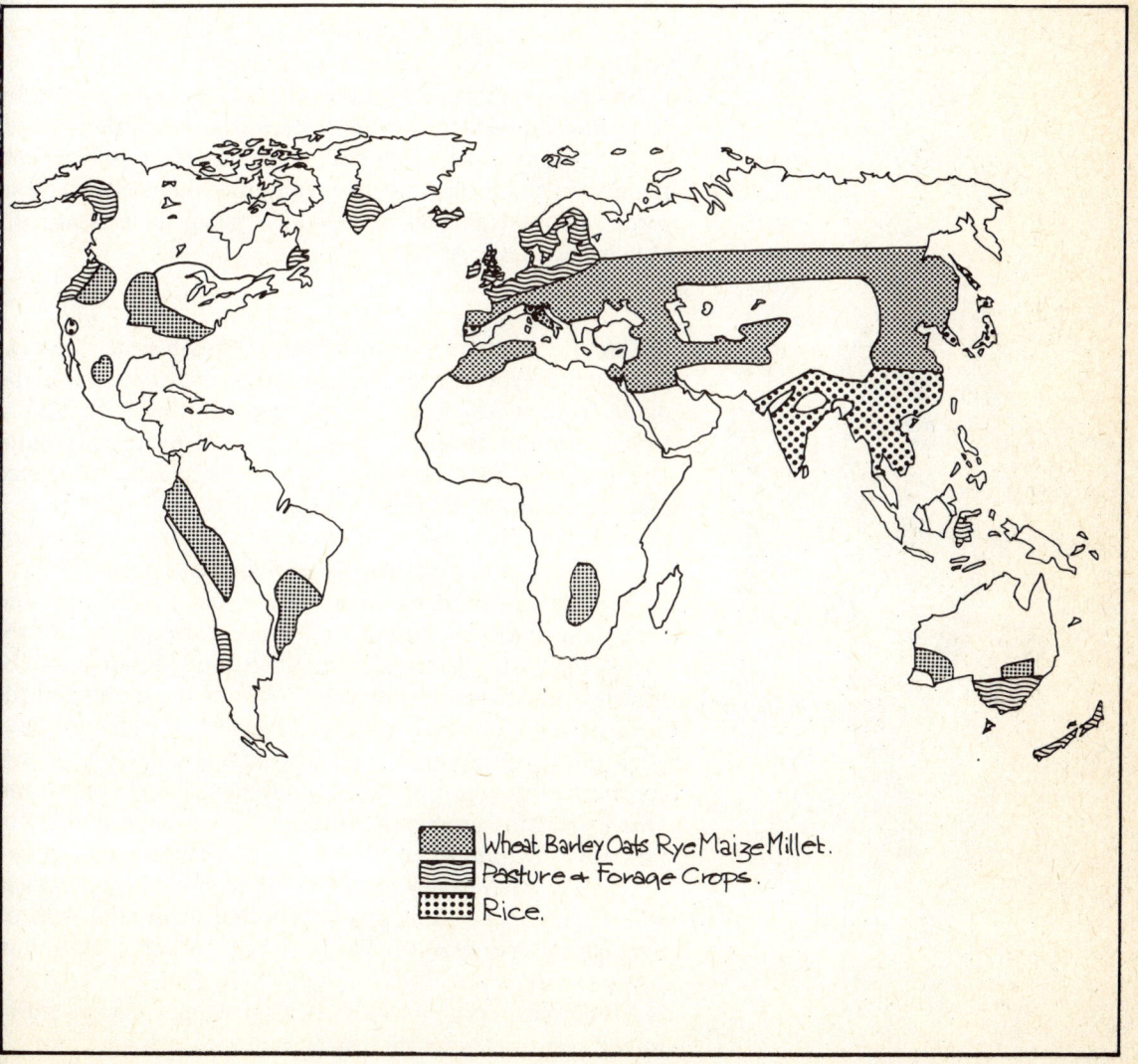

Wheat Barley Oats Rye Maize Millet.
Pasture & Forage Crops.
Rice.

cultivate the wild grain-bearing grasses that men decided to settle in one place long enough for crops to grow to seed-time, and to select for their settlement districts where the climate and the soil suited their primitive skills in agriculture.

Cereal crops have provided the staple food of most races or nations ever since those earliest settlements and the kind of grain that grows best in a given area has become the basis of the diet of people living in that area; for example, rice in eastern countries; wheat in Central Europe and later in the United States; maize in Central and South America; and rye, barley and oats in Northern Europe.

Nowadays all parts of the world are so closely linked by trade that the well-to-do countries can vary their diet almost at will. Many developing countries, however, still depend mainly on the foods that they can grow themselves and in some regions tradition makes only certain cereals acceptable in the diet.

Wheat

By far the most important cereal in British food is wheat because the type of bread eaten in this country can only be made from wheat flour. The reason for this is that only wheat contains enough of two important proteins, gliadin and glutenin, to make (with water) the elastic substance gluten, necessary to produce the crusty well-risen loaves that we like. There are different strains of wheat which vary in the amounts and qualities of protein they contain. Wheat with a high proportion of protein is termed 'strong' and that with a lower content or a poorer quality is termed 'weak' or 'soft'. Flour for making good bread must be milled from strong wheat; it must not be overheated in the drying which follows combine harvesting. It must not have been unduly weathered by rain delaying the harvest, and certainly it must not have sprouted in such wet conditions. Our uncertain summer weather does not make it easy for farmers in Britain to grow strong wheat such as that grown in Canada, where a dry summer with plenty of sun produces wheat with 14 per cent protein content compared with an average of 9 per cent for British wheat, which is classed as soft or weak.

Modern experiments with wheat-growing are now leading to the use of strains of seed-wheat with a higher protein

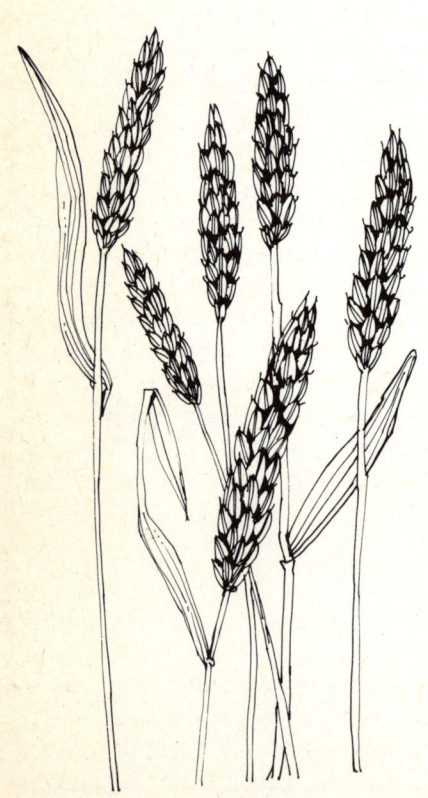

content, and to improvement in methods of cultivation. The bakery industry is also working to develop methods of making good bread from soft flour; one such method is the Chorley Wood Bread Process. By this process ascorbic acid is added to the dough which is worked very vigorously, of course mechanically, for a short time using a higher proportion of yeast than in older methods. The two industries together may in future make it possible for more bread to be made from homegrown wheat.

Around 3·5 million tons of wheat are grown in this country each year but of this only about 0·7 million tons is milled into flour for bread making for which purpose it is usually blended with strong Canadian wheat which makes up two-thirds of the required total. Of the rest of the home-grown wheat some 0·5 million tons is used as the soft flour needed for biscuit making, another 0·5 million for flour for cakes and household use, while 1·5 million tons is not milled as flour but is used for animal feeding, with some 0·2 million tons reserved as seed for the next year's crop. Pasta, that is macaroni and similar products, is made from a very hard wheat known as 'durum' which has an extra high proportion of protein.

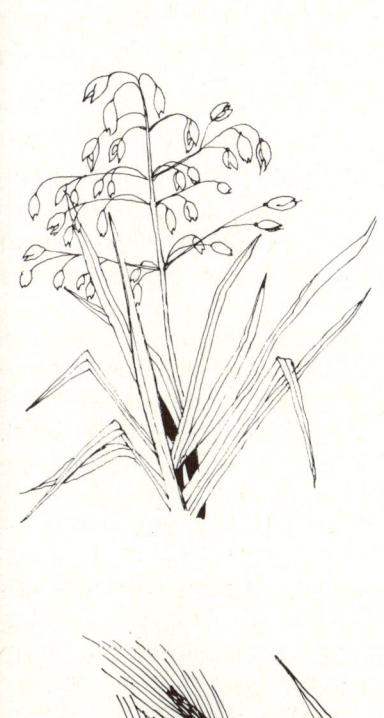

Oats

Oats will grow in conditions of climate and soil that are not suited to wheat and although they cannot be used for bread making they are excellent food for human beings and for animals. For our own food we use oats as porridge, breakfast cereals and oatcakes, and they have in the past been the staple food of parts of Scotland where they are still popular and where they grow well. Oats are valuable for animal feeding because they have a good proportion of fibre, which animals need to aid digestion, and the fairly high fat content gives a bloom to the coats of horses and young calves.

Barley

Barley is grown in all parts of Britain; it grows well in soil that is too poor for wheat growing. It is used mainly for animal feeding and for making malt, used in brewing beer and in the processes of the production of whisky. It is important in the modern feeding of young beef animals. A little barley is used for human food, for example as pearl barley.

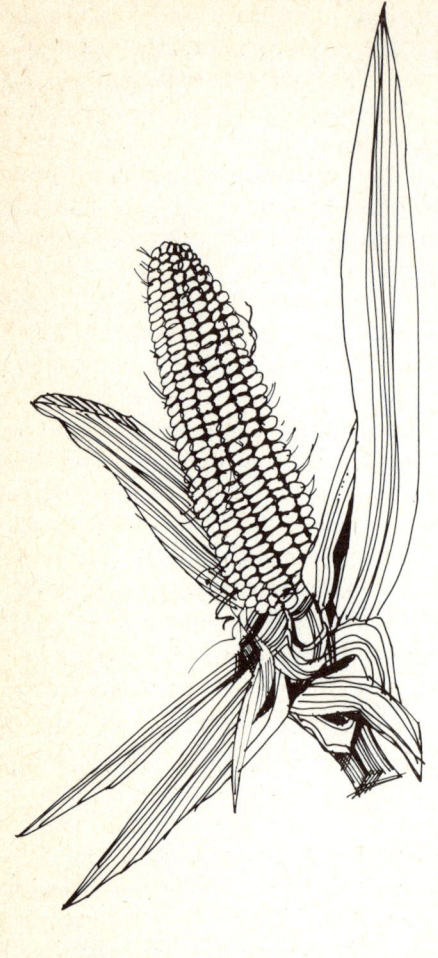

Rye

Rye is not grown or used a great deal in Britain. It i
another cereal which grows in soil and climate not suitabl
for wheat, it does best in a fairly hot, dry summer.

The demand for rye is growing as the popularity of ry
crispbread increases and the rye grown in Britain is parti
cularly suitable for this product. In the future more rye ma
be grown in this country so that it may replace some of tha
imported from Canada both for crispbread and as a substi
tute for maize in animal food. Rye bread, popular on th
Continent, can be bought in England; it usually has som
wheat flour mixed with rye to provide enough gluten.

Maize

Maize for 'indian corn' needs very hot weather to ripen it
Maize originated in South America, was later grown i
Central America and is now grown extensively in the Unite
States. It was brought to Europe by early Spanish explorer
and is grown now in Mediterranean countries.

Maize is used in this country for cornflour (a pure starch
for breakfast cereals, for cooking oil, for the manufactur
of margarine and as corn for animal food. For all thes
purposes it is imported and also as sweet corn as a vegetabl

For many years we have grown maize in Britain as gree
fodder or silage for cattle as it is a very good food for dair
cows. It is now being grown experimentally to ripen a
grain, in addition to silage, for animal feeding. The seed use
for this crop must be a hardy hybrid that will ripen early
It cannot withstand frost and it needs light, well-draine
soil. Given the right conditions it should be a useful crop fo
feeding cattle and other animals.

Rice

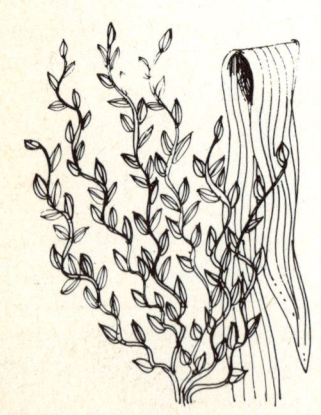

Rice cannot be grown in Britain as it needs a hot climate
with flooded fields for its start in life. It was first cultivated i
China, whence it was introduced to the whole continent o
Asia. The Romans brought it from Asia to Europe and i
the seventeenth century it was taken to the southern states o
America, so that now it is grown in southern Europe, part
of Africa and parts of the U.S.A. It is imported into Britai
from the United States, from Italy, China and Thailand
Many Asian countries need all the rice they can grow to fee
their own huge populations, whose staple food it still is.

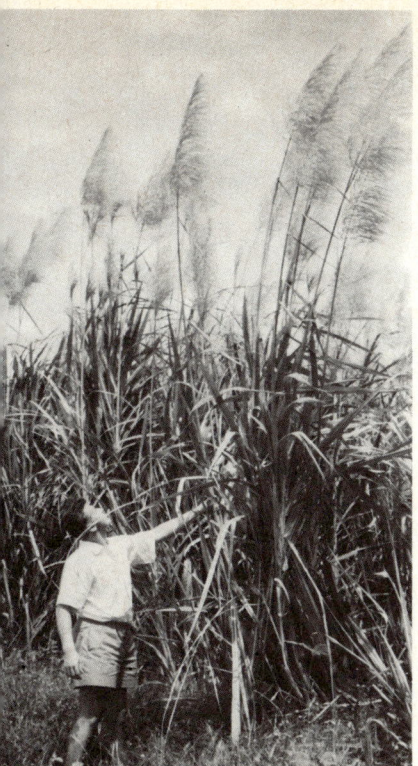

Sugar cane plantation

Cut sugar cane

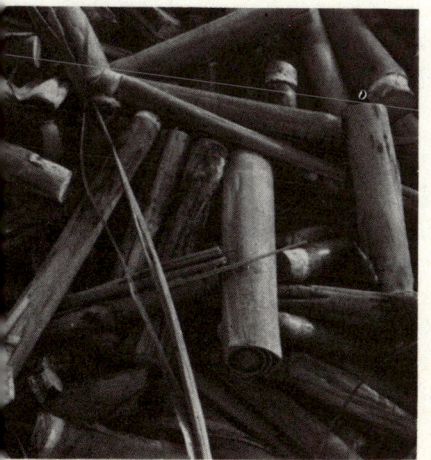

SUGAR

In Britain we eat a great deal of sugar—far too much according to dietitians and dentists—in fact about a hundredweight (50 kg) for each one of us each year! This, of course, includes sweets and the sugar used in drinks, biscuits, cakes, household cooking and preserving.

All plants contain some sugar, which they manufacture from carbon dioxide in the air, with the help of sunlight, by a process known as *photosynthesis*. To make it worth while to manufacture sugar commercially a plant must be chosen which stores a large amount of it. The first such plant, which we now call sugar cane, was seen growing in India by Darius, Emperor of Persia in 510 B.C. He called it 'the reed that makes honey without bees'. Later, Alexander the Great in the fourth century B.C. had it imported to the Mediterranean and from there its cultivation spread to Egypt, Persia, Arabia and North Africa. By the thirteenth century A.D. a little sugar was imported to England where very rich people only could afford it—the rest had to make do with honey.

By the sixteenth century sugar cane was being planted in the West Indies by the Spanish and Portuguese and, when Britain acquired Jamaica and other West Indian Islands, British sugar planters made large fortunes and sugar refineries were built in Britain. We still import a great deal of cane sugar from the West Indies.

Sugar cane can only grow in a tropical climate with plenty of water, either from heavy rainfall or frequent irrigation; such a climate occurs in Cuba, Brazil and Western Australia, as well as in the West Indies and in the Old World countries already named. Sugar cane is really an enormous grass growing to 12 or 15 feet high. It is harvested either by machines or by hand with a sharp heavy knife. It is stripped of leaves, which are used for cattle food, and hurried to the sugar mill where it is crushed by rollers, boiled to extract the sugar syrup, freed from impurities (that is any dissolved substances that are not pure sugar) and finally by most exactly timed and skilful treatment reduced to a brown, sticky mass of crystals mixed with syrup. By centrifugal force the crystals and syrup are separated to raw sugar and molasses. The molasses is used for making cattle food, yeast and rum. The fibrous part of the cane has already been removed for use as fuel for the

101

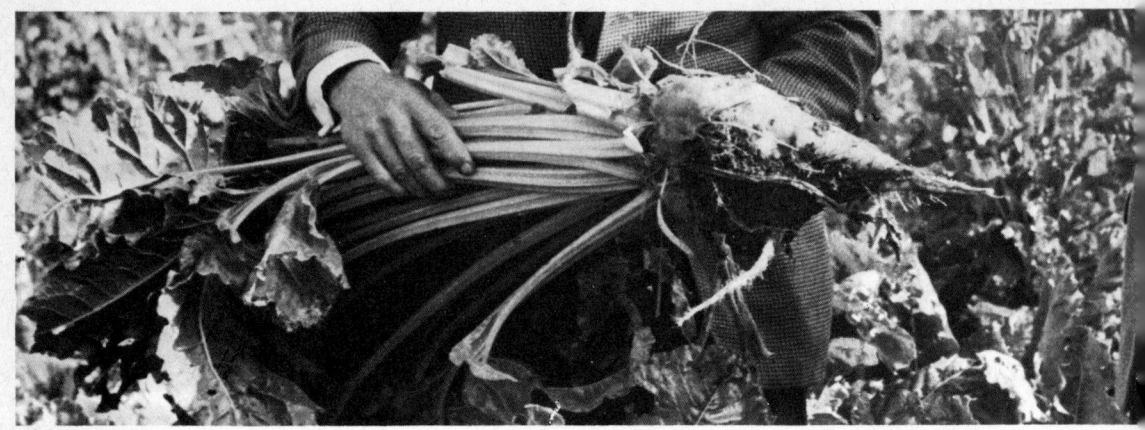

Sugar beet

boilers or for the making of paper and hardboard.

In Britain we grow one-third of all the sugar we consume but, as we obviously have not the right climate for sugar cane, we grow sugar beet instead, a plant which stores sugar in its roots. Experiments were made as early as 1832 to cultivate sugar beet which was already known in its wild form, but it was not until after the 1914–18 war that a sugar beet industry was successfully established.

The beet is grown in the Eastern Counties and the West Midlands of England. The seed is sown in spring and harvested in autumn by a combine that slices off the green tops and lifts the roots from the ground. The leafy tops are used for silage for cattle food. The sugar is now extracted by slicing the washed beet and soaking it in hot water to draw out the juice by *osmosis*. The process is simpler than that used for sugar cane as the beet being softer does not need rollers to crush it and also as many impurities remain trapped in the cell walls of the beet. The raw sugar and molasses are now prepared for refining; the pulp is used for cattle food, as is some of the molasses; the latter is greatly relished by cows in their silage or cattle-cake. Some of the molasses is used, not for rum, but for making industrial alcohol.

The refined sugar we can buy in several forms as granulated, caster, cube and, less refined, as various kinds of brown sugar and the syrup which will not crystallise readily, as golden syrup or black treacle. It is worth noting that chemically sugar from sugar cane and sugar beet is absolutely identical.

Things to do

1. Look out for agricultural shows in your area and there study the various breeds of cattle, sheep and pigs.
2. School will probably arrange farm visits, the Association of Agriculture can advise and can help to arrange these. If you can go on such a visit take note of arrangements for milking, of the kind of food and the method of distributing it to the cows, the method by which the milk is sent to the bottling plant and any other details of farm management.
3. If you can, also visit a market garden with glasshouses; an orchard; a farm growing sugar beet; an arable farm with grain drying arrangements.
4. Make a thorough study, backed up by visits, of any one or more topics dealt with in this chapter, for example: beef production, the dairy industry, the egg producing industry, the poultry industry, sheep rearing, wheat production and research, the bakery industry, market gardening, or any other that you can think of.

Further reading

PERRY, G. A. *Investigator's book of soils,* Blandford, Rural Studies, 1965.

BOLGER, F. J. *Animal husbandry,* Blandford Rural Studies, 1965.

GLEN, ANN. *Contemporary Scotland,* Heinemann, Educational books, 1969.

JOHNSON, RAYMOND. *Farms in Britain,* Macmillan, 1970.

ARCHER, D. M. *Science and Food Production,* E. J. Arnold, 1971.

WATERS, D. *Milk and maths,* National Dairy Council (undated).

NATIONAL DAIRY COUNCIL BOOKLETS: Churns and cheeses, 1970; Handbook of dairy foods, 1971; Breeds of cow—British dairy cows, No. 10.

PAMPHLETS FROM: British Egg Information Service; British Farm Produce Council; Apple and Pear Development Council; British Meat Services; Kellogs Ltd.—'The grains are great foods'; The Gas Council—'Cooking, gas and you'—Cereals, Meat, Poultry; T. Wall and Sons; British Sugar Bureau, 'White Gold', 1971; and many others.

6 Food All Over the World

THE HAVES AND THE HAVE NOTS

In previous chapters we have considered what food human beings need, how they can best use it and where some of the foods come from that we eat in Britain. So far we have been concerned with food in Britain, by world standards a reasonably well-off country and one that is technically and industrially advanced. If we now take a wider look at food supplies all over the world we shall see conditions in many countries that are very different from our own. There are countries in Africa, South and Central America, the Middle East, the Far East and Asia generally, where there is barely

Primitive farming in Africa

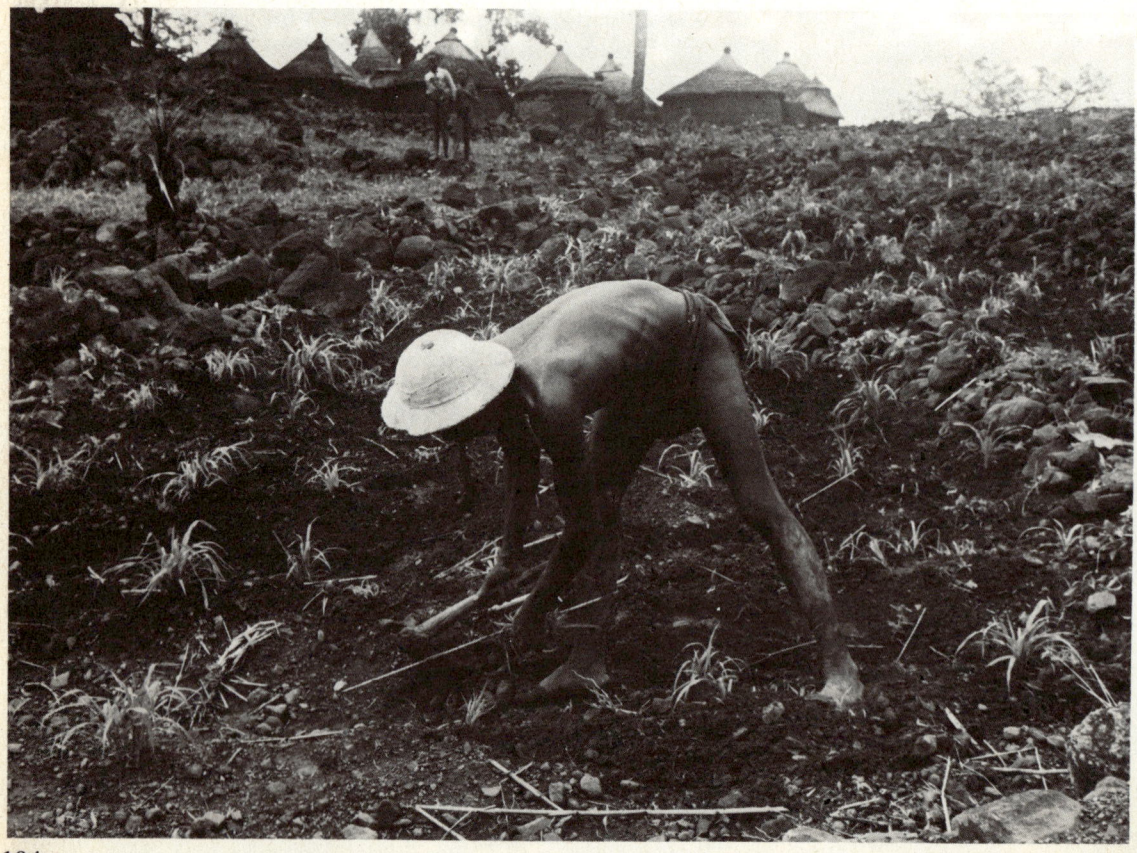

enough, and at times not nearly enough, food to satisfy the population. To such peoples it is not much use knowing how much food and what kind of food they need, they also need to find out how in the world to get it.

About three-quarters of the world's population is, in one way or another, chiefly concerned with producing food, either just for the subsistence of their own families or, on a larger scale, to help supply the whole community yet, in spite of this, a very large part of the world still remains hungry. Scientists who work with statistics applied to world conditions have prophesied that, by the year 2000, the population of the world will have increased so much that, even if the present steady improvement in food production continues, there will not be enough food for everyone. More optimistic experts points out that mankind, through thousands of years, has repeatedly met terrible problems and has managed to tackle and solve them. Nowadays technology is advancing so fast that new problems will, we hope, be solved by new methods.

At present there is enough food in the world to supply the whole world population with enough protein, calories and other essential nutrients if it could be shared out equally. In some countries, the 'developed' or well-to-do ones, many people eat more than they really need; they are accustomed to this level of nutrition and would feel deprived with less. In such countries some quite common diseases are mainly caused by over-eating while in poorer or developing countries more disease arises from malnutrition or under-nutrition.

Why is food not shared equally throughout the world? There are very many reasons and, without going into politics, some of the simple answers are that in developed countries the farmers who produce food need to make a living for themselves and for everyone who works for them. Countries which have enough food to sell some abroad have to earn money from export sales to run their own affairs. In times of disaster such as floods, earthquakes, droughts and other people's wars many countries do their best to send help in kind where it is needed, but this is only a temporary remedy. In normal times those countries which cannot produce enough food for their own use are also usually unable to export much of anything and therefore cannot afford to buy food abroad nor do they wish to live on gifts

SIZE OF FAMILIES

In the past,
half the children
died.

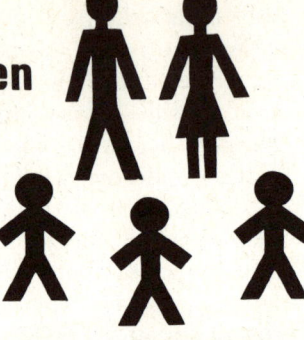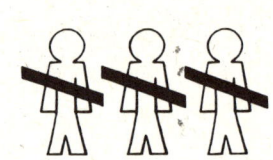

How many grandchildren ?

Today, with
better medicine,
nearly all
survive.

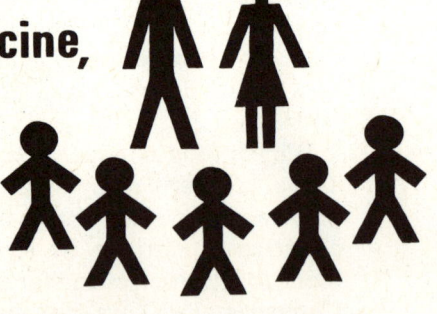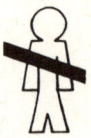

How many grandchildren ?

Prepared by Pictorial Charts Educational Trust for War on Want, London, W.5.

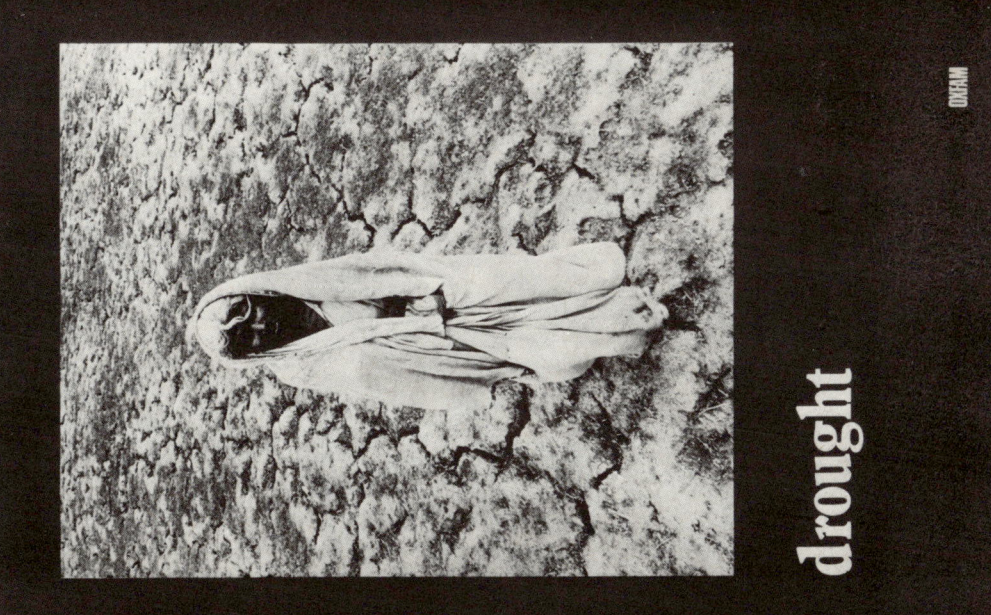

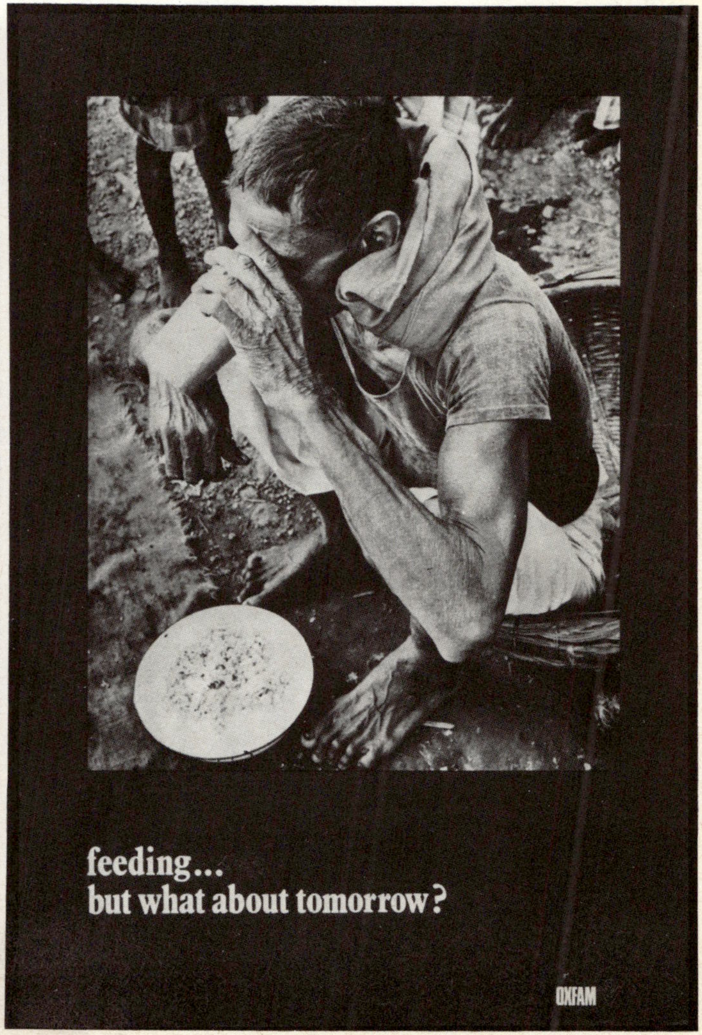

feeding...
but what about tomorrow?

OXFAM

drought

OXFAM

107

from wealthy neighbours. National dignity and independence are important. Another difficulty of sharing is that people are conservative about food and cannot accept as edible food which is strange to them; for example, to Asian peoples who live largely on rice wheat is very odd and is therefore rejected.

THE CAUSES OF MALNUTRITION

Malnutrition is a condition in which the body does not receive the right proportion of all the nutrients; the nutrients in short supply are usually proteins, vitamins and minerals. Because starchy foods are usually the most plentiful and because they satisfy hunger they are not usually lacking in the diet. If food is so scarce that all nutrients are in short supply *undernutrition* is the result; the extreme of this is starvation.

Undernourished African cattle in a dry season

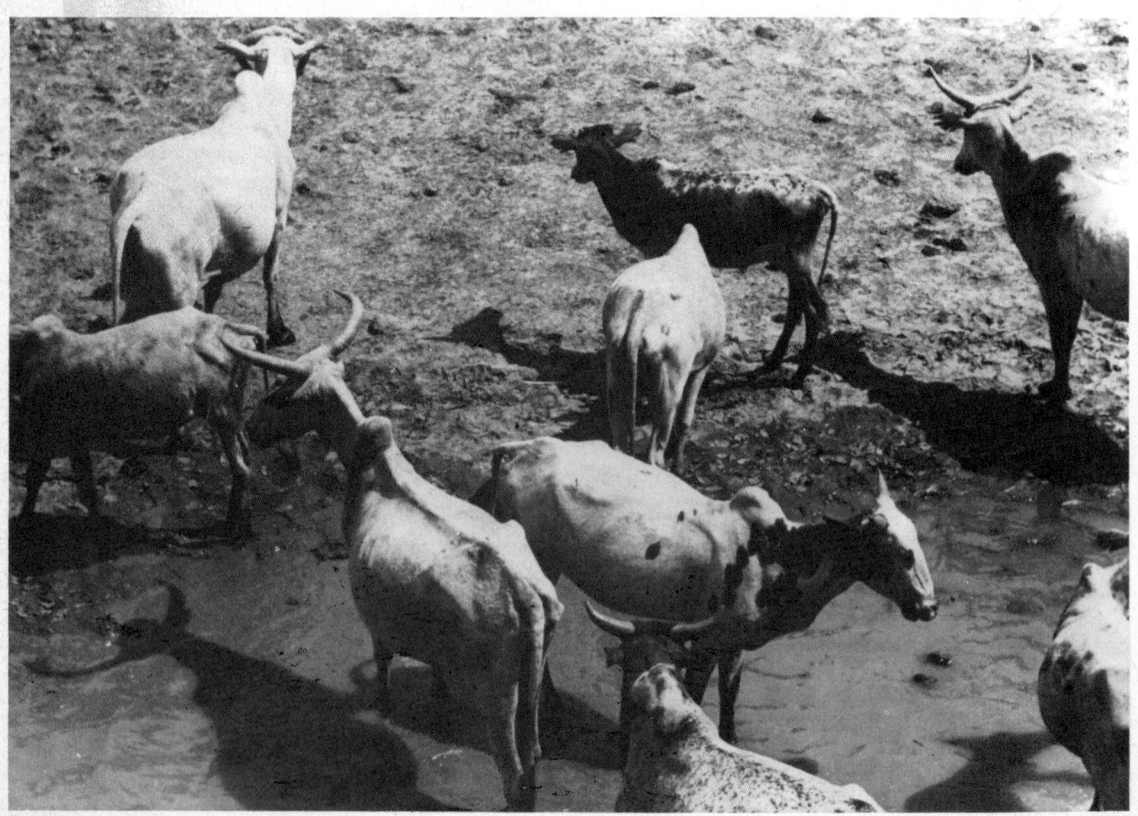

There are many causes for the malnutrition of any group of people. The chief cause is that they just cannot produce enough of the right foodstuffs because they have not the knowledge of agriculture nor the right tools; because the soil is poor; because there is not enough water to irrigate the crops; because insect pests destroy the crop and weaken any animals they keep and because, if they are undernourished or malnourished, they have not the energy to improve their farming. Other causes are the lack of money or goods to barter for tools, good seeds or good breeds of livestock and the need to raise a little money by growing cash crops of such things as tobacco, cotton, coffee or cocoa, leaving too little land for food crops. Sometimes the food itself may be sold in the towns, leaving too little for the family; sometimes the easiest crops to grow and harvest replace those that require more skill and energy, for example, cassava (a starch root from which we get tapioca) is grown in some districts of Africa instead of millet which has much more protein and more vitamins. Sometimes the younger men of the village go to the towns to get work, leaving only women and old men to work in the fields.

When families move from a primitive country village to a town, in their strange, new surroundings they may miss the familiar foods they grew at home and, having for the first time to buy food, they are often unable to choose wisely. The cheapest or the most attractive-looking, or the best advertised, are perhaps chosen. They do not necessarily contain the right nutrients; too often they have a low protein content and maybe too much starch and sugar.

Even where there is enough food of the right kind for the whole community there may be certain rules and beliefs governing the diet of some section of the family, most usually women, girls and little children. For example, in some parts of Africa, women and girls are forbidden to drink milk, which is supposed to prevent them from ever having babies; in villages in parts of Central America and in the Far East, although chickens, eggs and meat are plentiful they are thought to be quite unsuitable foods for young children; sometimes fish is also denied to children; in some districts in India expectant mothers are not allowed eggs, and some African tribes will not eat fish even when their main source of protein from wild game animals is no longer available. In addition there is also a widespread belief that

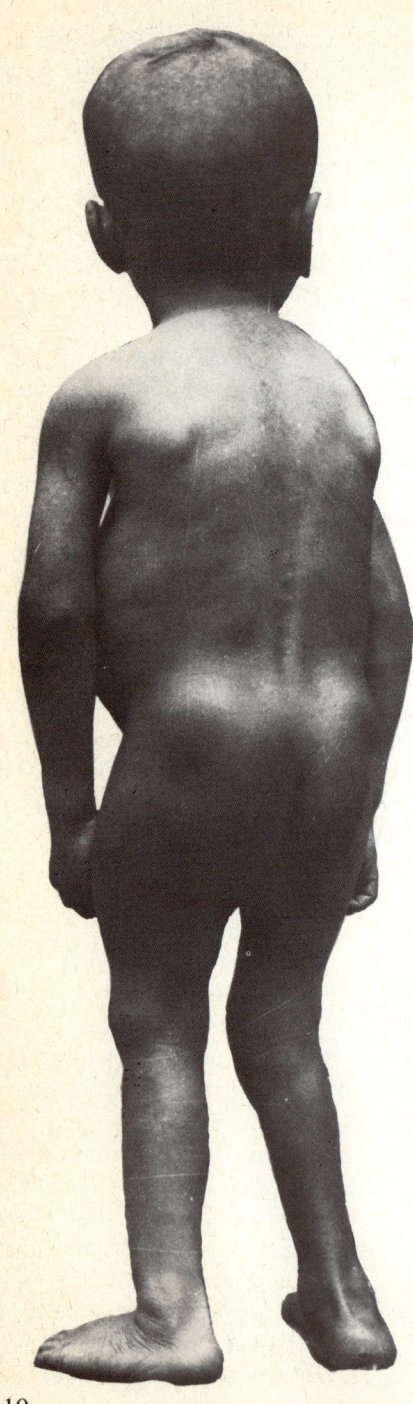

men and boys, being originally the warriors and hunters, must have the best food (and that means most of the protein foods) while the women, girls and tiny children make do with what is left.

In most of the developing countries two-thirds of the population is made up of children and their mothers. With the restrictions mentioned above it follows that where food is scarce many thousands of children suffer from serious malnutrition and they and their mothers contract deficiency diseases that are rarely found nowadays in the better-off countries. While young babies are still breast fed they remain healthy because even a poorly nourished mother can usually provide enough milk; it is when they are weaned that their diet is liable to become inadequate, as it is often by custom mainly semi-liquid, starchy foods with no fruit or vegetable and very little protein. So the very important sections of a race—the babies who have to grow up to be the adults of the future and the mothers who are expected to bear more babies—are the first to suffer from malnutrition.

Some of the diseases which are caused by malnutrition are *rickets* and *osteomalacia*, diseases of the bones which occur when vitamin D, calcium and phosphorus are lacking (vitamin D may be lacking even in a sunny climate because it may be customary for babies to be kept well covered up and indoors); *beri-beri* and *pellagra,* which affect the nerves and the heart as well as producing other symptoms (both are caused by lack of the vitamin B complex) and *xerophthalmia,* an eye disease caused by lack of vitamin A.

Still another deficiency disease, this one caused by shortage of protein is *kwashiorkor,* the name given to it in one West African language. Weaned babies and children up to five years old are the victims of this disease; they do not grow or gain weight, they are peevish and miserable, their bodies swell although their limbs may be pitifully weak and thin, they often suffer from sickness and diarrhoea and their hair is bleached in patches. Even if the unfortunate infants do not die of these diseases, which they often do, they are much more likely to fall prey to other diseases such as measles or whooping-cough; they do not develop mentally or physically as well as well-fed children, and they have a poor chance of growing up into vigorous men and women. Unfortunately illness is not always understood as being curable or in any way caused by wrong feeding, it is

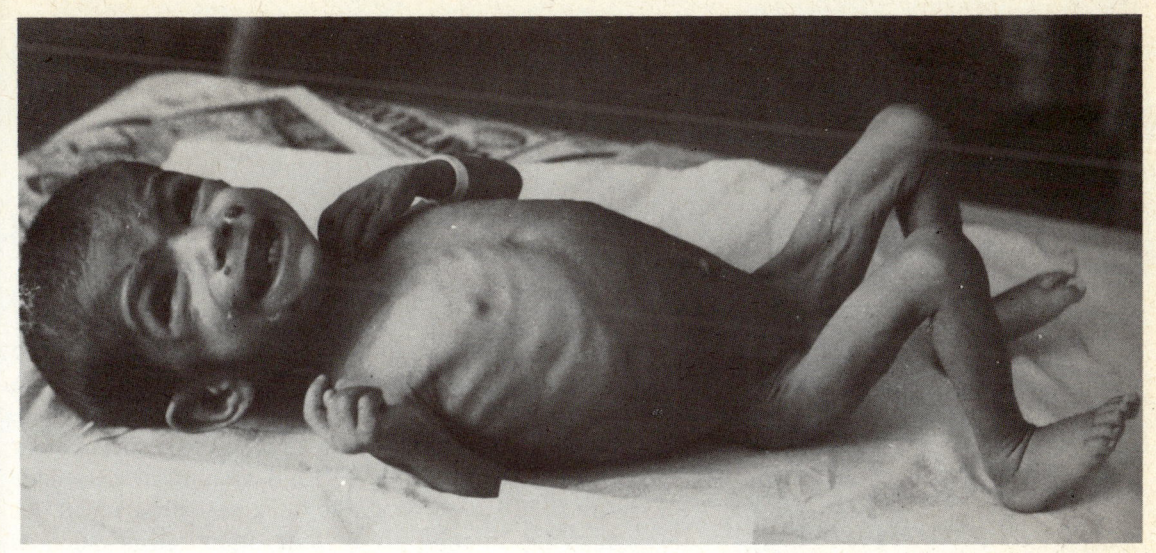

Left *A child with rickets*
Above *A typical case of malnutrition*
Right *The same child after
treatment—ten months later.*

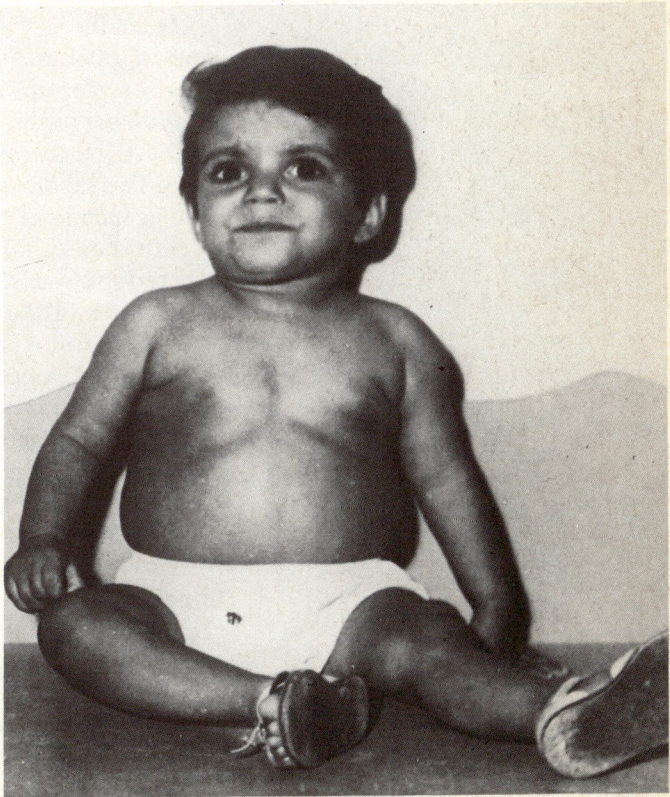

often thought to be due to the spite of evil spirits and only to be dealt with by a witch doctor who can drive away the spirits by his magic.

THE REMEDIES

As sharing out the food supplies of the world is not practical nor possible the best way to set about fighting malnutrition and undernutrition is to share knowledge of agriculture, technology, science in any branch bearing on food, pest control and, of course, nutrition. Information should be made available to all countries with the aim of enabling them to produce all the food of which their land is capable, not forgetting their lakes, rivers and sea coast. *The United Nations* has undertaken work with these aims in view since the end of the 1939–45 war. The work has been carried out through many different groups and organisations such as U.N.I.C.E.F., the United Nations Children's Fund; W.H.O., the World Health Organisation; F.A.O., the Food and Agriculture Organisation; and P.A.G., the Protein Advisory Group. The work has grown steadily and it has to include the raising of enough money from member nations of the U.N. to carry out research, teaching and practical help. This kind of aid is also undertaken by many voluntary bodies such as Oxfam, and the Save the Children Fund.

As a start U.N.I.C.E.F. sent dried skim milk to countries where food was scarce to be given to children to improve their diet a little. This was only a stop-gap; the real work began with making exact calculations of how much food was needed for people to work and thrive in various climates and various types of work and in making periodic surveys of the state of agriculture all over the world so that advice could be given to the governments of different regions as to the best way of dealing with their food problems and of making the most of their own resources. Next came help in the form of money for the training of people in the developing countries to become experts in many branches of agriculture and for setting up field projects and carrying out research. Where food itself was sent it was used as part of wages for work.

Wealthy countries were encouraged to lend money, as investment, to the developing countries to enable them to buy the fertilisers, seed, pesticides, tools, breeding animals

Right *Plague of locusts*

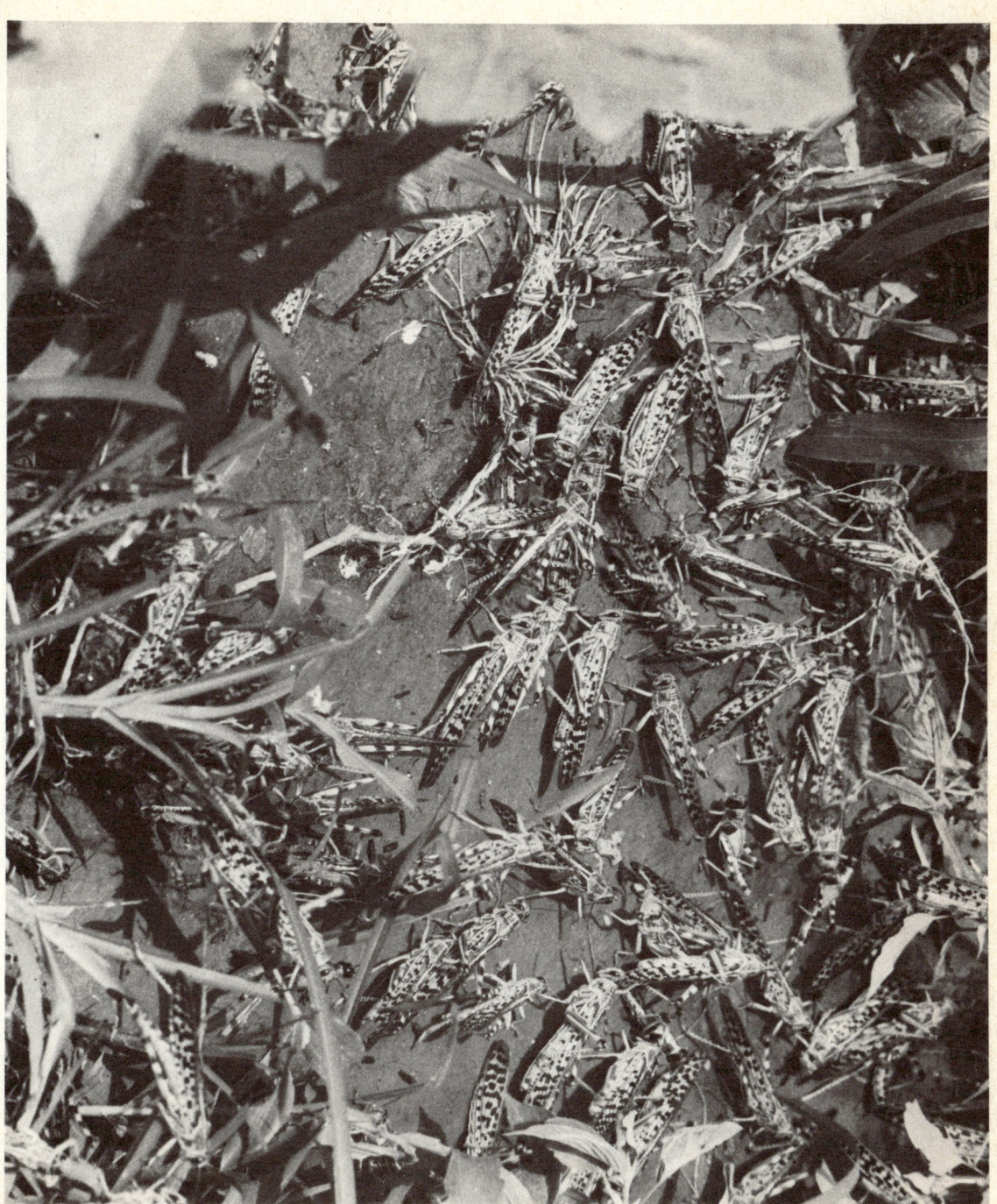

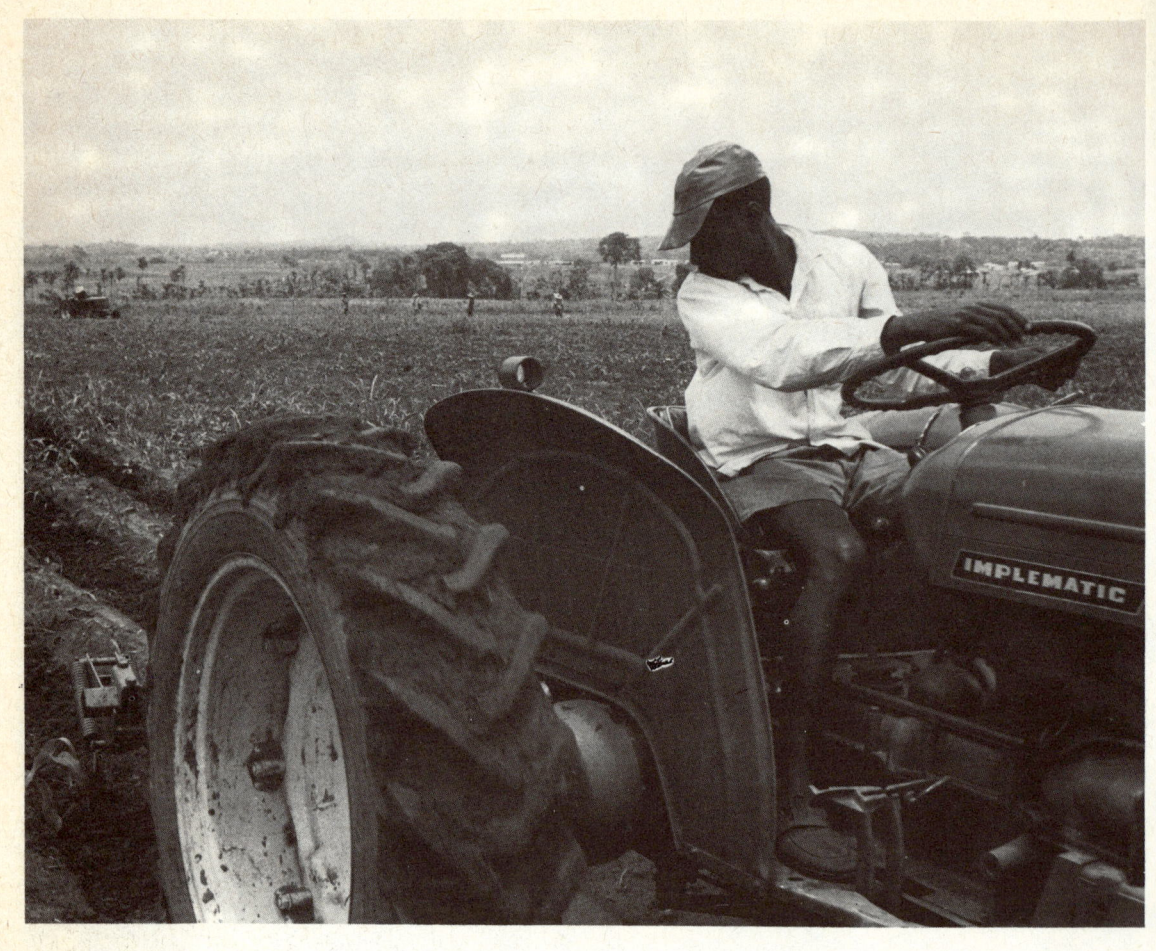

Modernised farming in Africa

or whatever they needed to improve food production. As well as direct help for agriculture it was usually necessary to give advice and practical help for the development of trade in other natural resources of the country, such as timber, hides and cotton, and the development of local industry.

The practical work includes control of pests such as locusts, which in their vast swarms can destroy every green crop for miles, and tsetse fly, which causes disease in men and cattle—sleepy sickness in men and often death for cattle. Irrigation schemes have been established in many parts of the world to store water, to cut irrigation canals and dig deep wells. Some desert land has been reclaimed and everywhere methods of improving the yield and the quality of crops have been studied. Increasing harvests of grain crops is of no use unless the grain can also be stored till the next harvest, so granaries have been built that can keep out animal and insect vermin which in the past have destroyed a large part of the food intended for human beings.

PROTEIN SHORTAGE

One of the most urgent problems has been the shortage of protein foods in the developing countries. Whereas in prosperous countries the average amount of protein each person eats in a day may be as high as 85 g, the average amount in poorer countries is 57 g, which means that many people get much less than that. Most of the protein in the developing countries comes from grain crops, so research is being carried out to increase the protein content of, for example, rice, millet and wheat. Encouragement is given

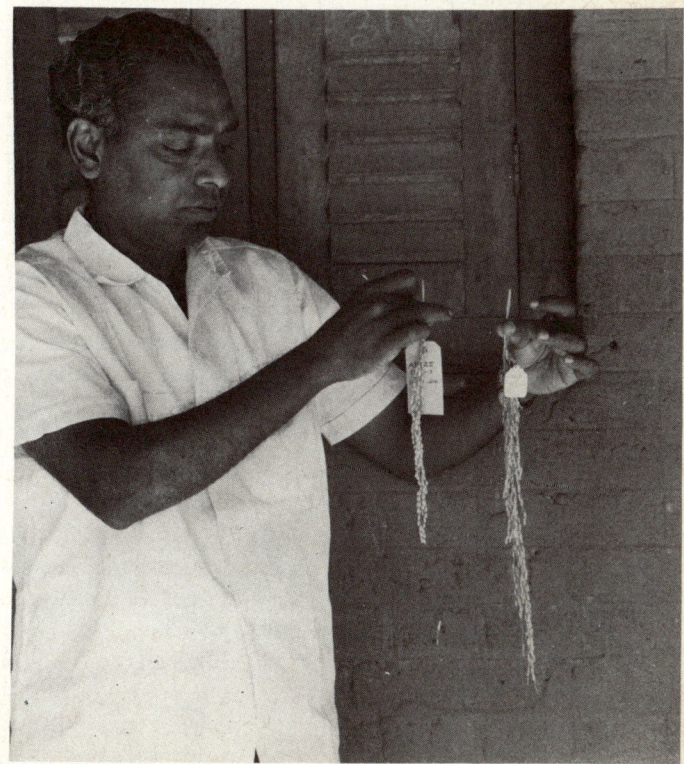

Comparing modern high yielding variety of rice with an earlier type

to the growing of cereals instead of starchy root crops such as yams and cassava, and where possible the inclusion of pulse crops (peas, beans and lentils), and in particular soybean, which has a high proportion of protein very like animal protein.

Animal protein is more easily converted to human protein than is that of plants but it is more expensive and often takes longer to produce, so, as well as trying to improve the breeding of cattle for beef and milk, F.A.O. has been encouraging the development of poultry, pork (where religion allows it) and fishery industries. If animals are to be kept successfully they must, of course, be properly fed, so attention also has to be given to improving grazing lands and to growing supplementary feeding stuffs for cattle.

Many governments of developing countries have schemes to distribute dried milk to children who are undernourished either at school or to their mothers if they are too young for school, but some countries cannot afford to do this without help from F.A.O. and other international agencies. Another way of ensuring that children, particularly in towns, can have enough protein in their diet is the manufacture of food mixtures made from ingredients grown in the country, with a reasonably high protein content but probably with additions of amino acids, vitamin A and calcium. Such a food mixture has to be made to a formula and produced in hygienic conditions, it is then packaged attractively and sold at a low price or distributed free to children in need of extra food. It is in a powder form that can be used in the normal diet of the country, perhaps in a thin gruel or in a porridge or in any baking. Such a product has to be made popular by advertising and it is used a great deal in schools where it is liked by most children. As a few examples:
Brazil makes Fortifex from maize and soybean,
Central America makes Incaparina from maize and cotton seed or soybean;
Britain and the Congo make Protone from maize, skim milk powder and yeast;
Nigeria makes Ariac from ground nuts and skim milk powder;
India makes Lac-tone from ground nuts, skim milk powder, wheat and barley;
East Africa makes Supro from maize or barley, yeast and skim milk powder;

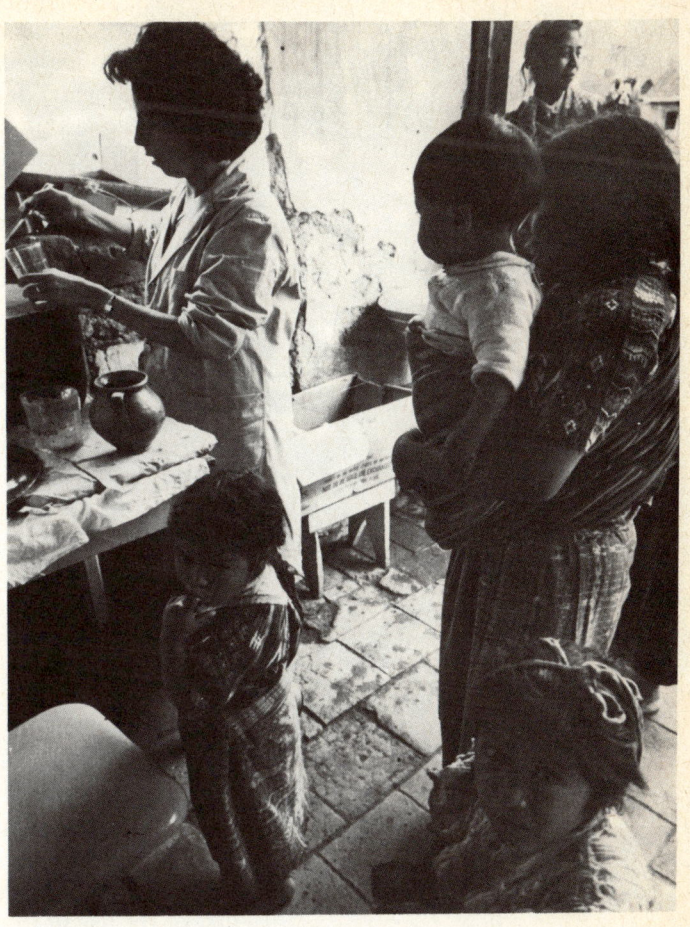

Distributing incaparina in Guatemala

there are others in other parts of the world. All have additions of amino acids, vitamins and calcium.

Little children when fed regularly on one of these mixtures can recover quickly from serious under nutrition including kwashiorkor.

A further development in the campaign to increase the protein supply of the world is the amount of research now being made into producing from vegetable proteins foods which can look and taste like meat or like dried skim milk. Soybean protein is converted to a liquid which is forced through fine tubes to set as fibres in a mass that closely resembles a pale coloured meat such as veal or chicken; or the liquid may be solidified in a granular form to look like

117

dried minced meat. It is carefully flavoured to taste like meat as well as to look like it, and can easily be cooked, usually with added water or sauce. These products are already being used by the catering trade and are available in special shops for sale to the general public. The idea of making a vegetable food (which vegetarians have enjoyed for years) appear like meat is that we are used to eating meat and will probably accept more easily such a 'reproduction' than we would the obviously vegetable original. In order to make the food go round in the rapidly increasing world population it may be necessary to increase vegetable crops rather than meat production because although all meat animals live on vegetable foods it takes some four tons of their food to produce one ton of meat.

The imitation dried milk is made by complicated processes from the protein in green leaves, in other words, by doing the work of the dairy cow. Several forms of vegetable 'milk' in powder form, including some made from soybean flour, have been on sale in 'health food' shops for years.

Another way of increasing the protein supply of the world is to produce protein of a single cell variety by allowing yeasts to grow on the waste from oil refineries; several experimental plants and one commercial plant are producing protein in this way for animal feeding. Certain bacteria (not the kinds that cause disease) can do the same work successfully and some fungi and algae (a kind of seaweed) have been tried, but not as yet with very good results. It is suggested that in the future protein of this kind may be grown for use in food for human beings.

EDUCATION

Just as these new methods of producing some of our food seem odd to us, and perhaps not very attractive, so do the ideas of F.A.O. and other campaigning agencies seem odd and not always immediately attractive to peoples in developing countries. For this reason another vitally important aspect of the work of getting the whole world properly fed is education. The people who really need to be educated in good feeding are the mothers who select the food and prepare meals for their families. Unfortunately they may not particularly want to be educated, their husbands may not want them educated either, and in any case

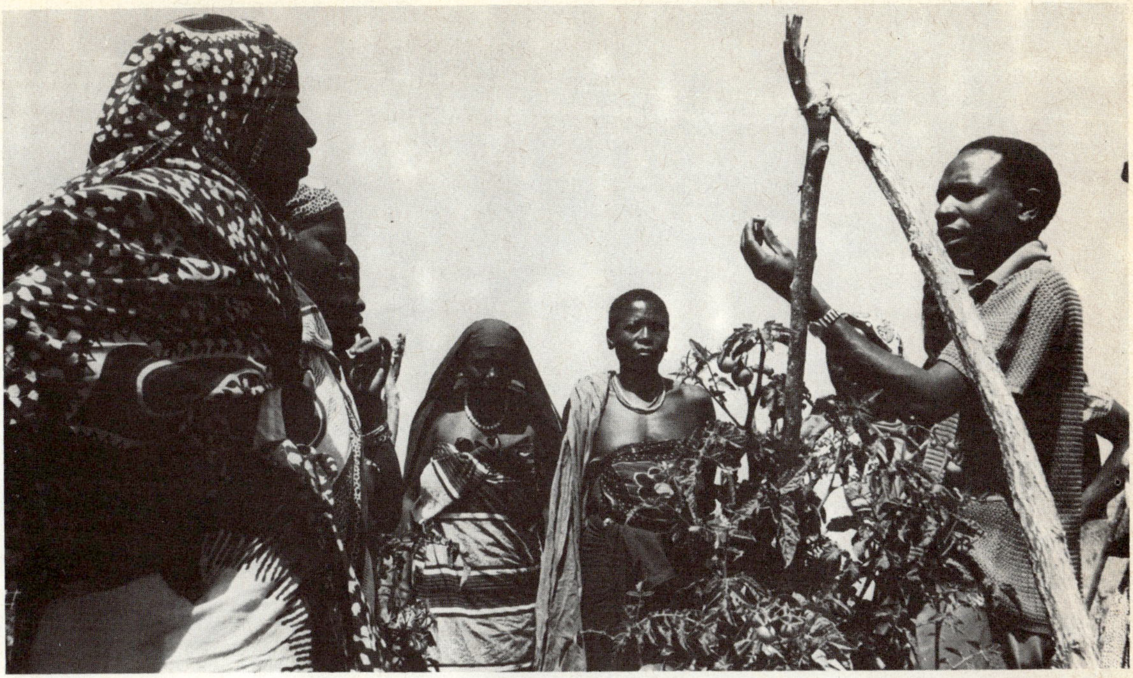

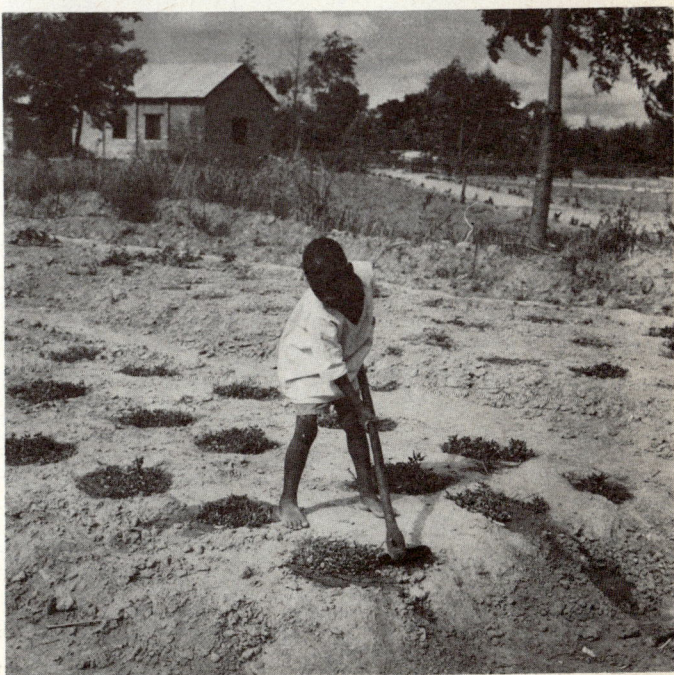

Teaching nutrition in Tanzania

Schoolboy learning to grow vegetables in Tanzania

119

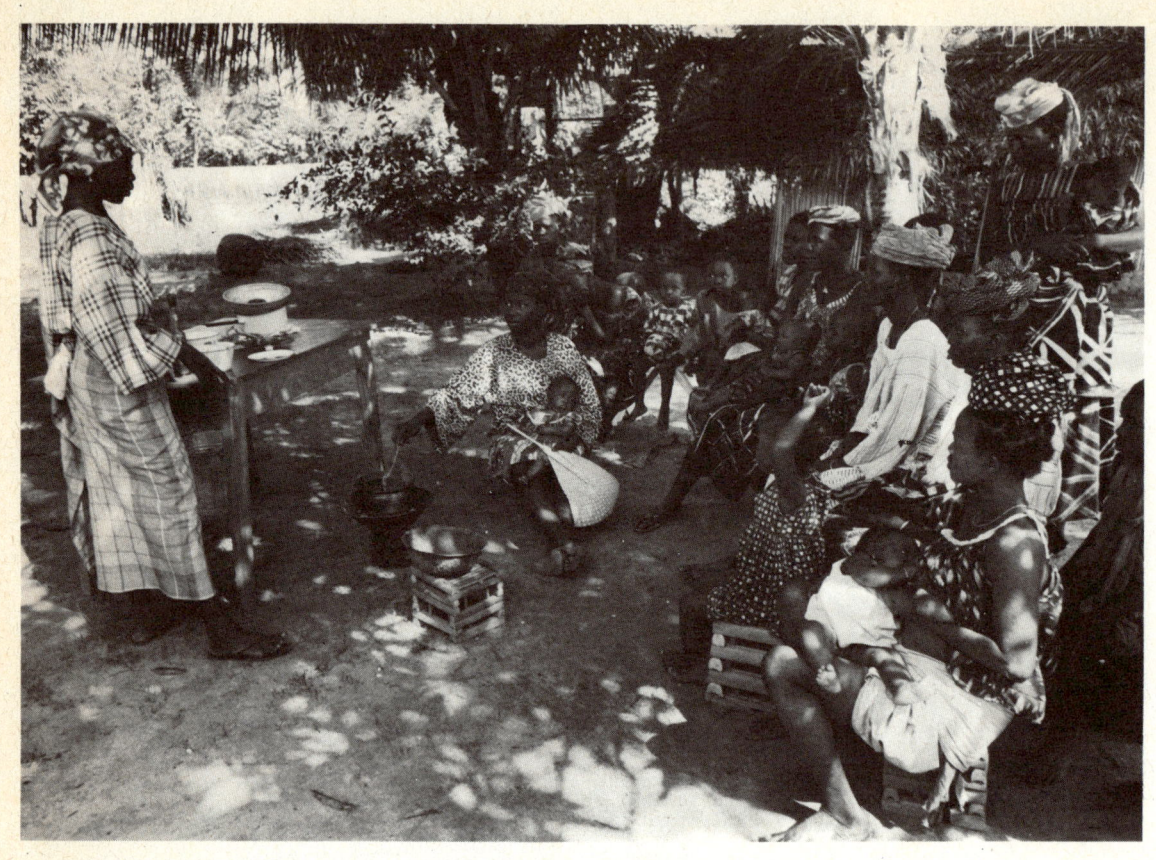

Teaching African mothers in Dahomey how to prepare food.

they may be busy. The teacher then has some problems. He or she must, of course, know the subject very well, must know how to teach and how people learn, and also how to persuade everyone in the community that understanding about food is a good thing. Often the programme of teaching nutrition grows from showing that good meals are making children healthier and happier, in other words from practical help in feeding, growing better crops and looking after domestic animals. Above all the teacher has to know and understand the way the community lives, what its food habits are and, if those habits are changing, how and why they are changing. Teaching may be given to men as well as women; often an understanding of what food the family needs can be fitted easily into help with local agriculture and a father may then encourage his wife in her efforts to do

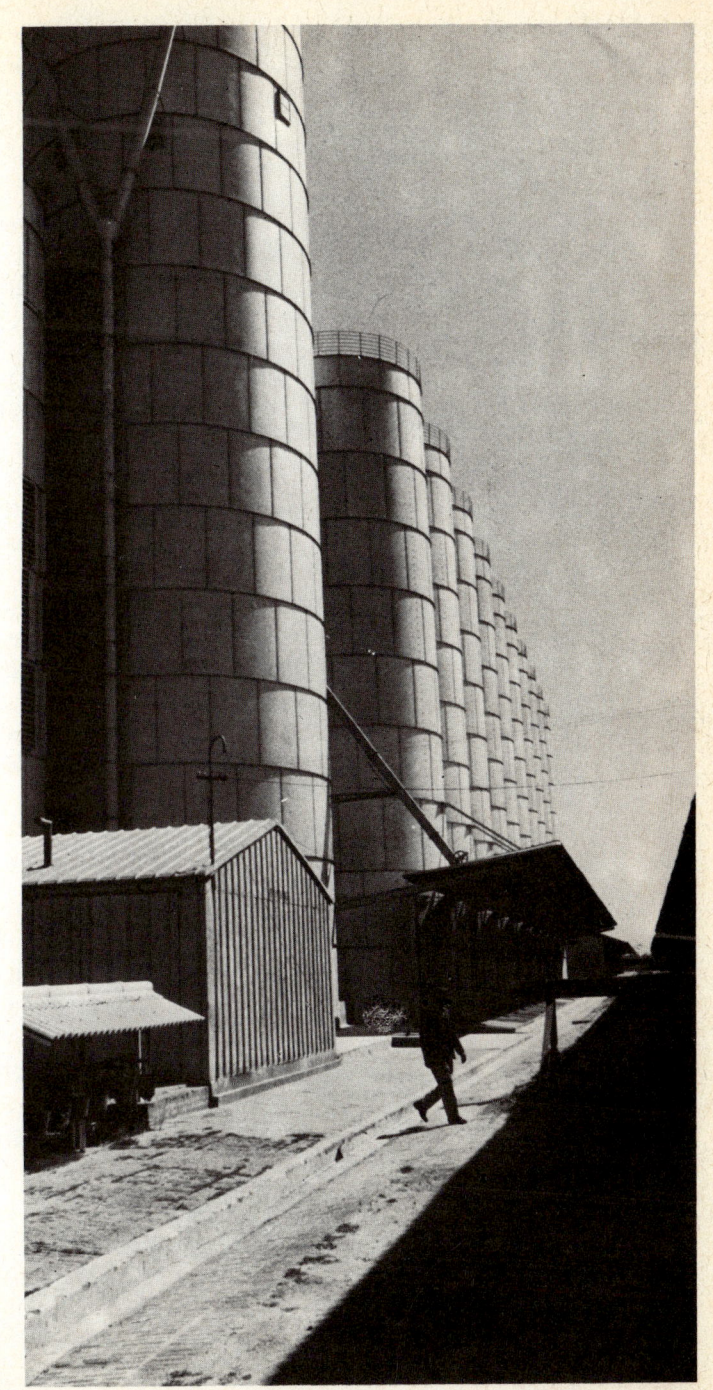

Modern grain silo in India.

the best for the family. It has also been found that education is accepted better from someone who normally works in the district such as the village school teacher, a health visitor or someone known in the village who has been away to learn about nutrition and/or agriculture and how to make it interesting and important to his friends and neighbours. One sure way of spreading a knowledge of nutrition is by teaching the children.

This kind of education needs a great deal of organisation and the Department of Education will deal with the training of teachers; the Departments of Agriculture and of Health will contribute expert knowledge; a Department of Food may help to see that the right food is available; there may also be Departments of Social Welfare or of National Planning and all these bodies will contribute to the whole programme for the country. Above all a Department of Finance will have to raise and grant the money and the Head of Government will have to approve and then to encourage everyone. Through all this complicated organisation foreign help, from such bodies as F.A.O. and kindred groups, is still vitally important, as it is from their experts that the scientific and technical knowledge comes. Finally, however, it is the people working at the 'grass roots' who have to prove that everyone in the world can be properly fed.

Things to do

1. Look in local shops for foods from India, Africa, West Indies, etc., vegetables, groceries, fish.
2. Try to make up a mixture as near to Incaparina etc., from foods that can be bought in this country. A health food shop may help. Perhaps school may help with purchase. Having made the mixture try making it into a pleasant drink or porridge.

Further reading

F.A.O., *Learning Better Nutrition,* 1971 (in print)
F.A.O., *Education and Training in Nutrition,* 1967, in print 1970.
F.A.O., *Child Care,* in print 1971.
Oxfam publications.

Miss Williams' Cookery Book, Longman. 4th Edition 1972.

STAMP, ELIZABETH. *The Hungry World,* Crossroads Series, E. J. Arnold, revised edition 1972.

LAWRY, J. H. *World Population and Food Supply,* Edward Arnold, 1970.

CHADWICK, LEE. *Seeds of Plenty in a Hungry World* (The World We Are Making), Methuen, 1968.

HARVEY, D., and MERRY, M. *People Poverty and Wealth* (Series—Certificate Topics in Geography), Collins, 1972.

MABEY, RICHARD. *Food,* Penguin Education, Connexions, 1972.

Index

Fat, 16, 20
Fibrous food, 21
Fish, 12, 18, 46, 47, 56, 87–91
Fruit, 12, 18, 95
Fuel, 20

Geese, 76
Glasshouses, 94
Gourmet menu, 18th century, 10
Gourmets, 11
Grapefruit, 12, 19
Green vegetables, 18, 19
Growth, 13, 27

Halibut, 16, 17
Ham, 12, 73
Health, 11, 31
Heat, 20
Herrings, 13, 15, 17
Home freezing, 57
Home production, 65
Homogenisation, 82
Honey, 12

Ice cream, 30
Imports, 64
Impulse buying, 41
Instant whips, 30
Iron, 15, 29, 31
Irrigation, 113

Jam, 12
Jelly, 30
Joule, 25

Kidney, 15, 18
Kwashiorkor, 110, 117

Lamb, 69
Lemons, 12, 19
Lentils, 12
Lettuce, 15, 19, 56
Line fishing, 89

Liver, 13, 15, 16, 17, 18
Livestock, 65
Local shop, 39
Locusts, 113

Mackerel, 13
Maize, 100
Malnutrition, 108
Margarine, 12, 16, 17
Markets, 41
Meats, 12, 23, 30, 34, 35
Meat, 12, 16, 46, 55, 66–73
Menu, choice of, 11
Metabolism, basal, 20
Milk, 12, 15, 17, 18, 30, 45, 80–7
Milking, 81
Millet, 109, 115
Minerals, 15
Molasses, 101, 102
Monosodium glutamate, 55
Mutton, 69

Niacin, 18
Nutrients, 13, 27
Nuts, 12

Oatmeal, 15, 18
Oats, 12, 99
Oil, 20, 49
Old people, 32, 61
Oranges, 12, 19
Osteomalacia, 110
Oxygen, 16

Packet soups, 30
P.A.G., 112
Pasta, 56, 99
Pasteurisation, 82
Pastry, 12, 56
Peas, 12, 16, 17
Pellagra, 110
Perishable food, 45
Phosphorus, 15, 17

125